ANABOLIC STEROIDS:
Altered States

James E. Wright, Ph.D.
(dward)

Virginia S. Cowart

F

COOPER
PUBLISHING
GROUP

RC
1230
W73
1990c

c.1

Library of Congress Cataloging in Publication Data:

WRIGHT, JAMES E., 1946 -
COWART, VIRGINIA S., 1937 -

ANABOLIC STEROIDS: ALTERED STATES

Cover Design: Gary Schmitt
Copy Editor: Kendal Gladish
Manufactured by: Cushing-Malloy, Inc.

Library of Congress Catalog Card number: 90-82102

ISBN: 1-884125-03-4

Printed in the United States of America by Cooper Publishing Group,
701 Congressional Blvd., Suite 340, Carmel, IN 46032

10 9 8 7 6 5 4

Dedications

To Jim and Jesse
J.W.

To David and Lark
V.C.

Foreword

While most attention has focused on the abuse of anabolic-androgenic steroids at the elite athlete level, what I call "the silent epidemic" has spread into the nation's high schools to a very alarming degree. Several studies have placed the incidence of anabolic-androgenic steroid use among male senior high school students at 6 to 7 percent. Figures as high as 11 percent of eleventh grade boys using steroids have been reported. In absolute terms, this means that between 250,000 and 500,000 high school students have used anabolic-androgenic steroids. More disturbing is the fact that approximately 40 percent have used five or more cycles, and approximately 40 percent began using steroids before the age of 16.

Why do high school students take these drugs? As expected, the majority are participants in school athletics and use them to enhance performance. But as many as a third of the male users are not involved in sports and take these drugs to enhance their appearance or masculinity.

There have been only a few surveys among the male college population and they show an estimated 2 percent usage. However, if we look at male college athletes, we find a more disturbing figure of between 5 and 17 percent.

The steroid problem is not restricted to males. As many as 1 to 2 percent of senior high school girls are users. Between 3 and 5 percent of Olympic and professional female athletes have admitted using them during their careers.

These figures all clearly support my claim that there is a "silent epidemic."

While I support controlling the production and sale of abused drugs, that is not the sole answer. In fact, we must be mindful that controlling the production of pharmaceutical grade anabolic-androgenic steroids carries with it the risk of increasing the availability of illicitly manufactured drugs. We must reduce the demand along with the supply.

Anabolic-androgenic steroids are important drugs that should remain available to the practicing physician, even though there are only a few medical conditions for which they are prescribed. They are used as hormonal replacement therapy for male patients, to manage certain blood disorders and cancers, and to treat a relatively rare inherited skin condition.

More research on the epidemiology of anabolic-androgenic steroid abuse and the health consequences of that abuse is needed. We must take definitive steps to arrest the further spread of this epidemic.

Anabolic Steroids: Altered States is one such definitive step to help fill the information void. Authoritatively written and easy to read, it presents the facts about anabolic-androgenic steroids as we know them.

Gary I. Wadler, M.D.

Acknowledgments

Both of us owe much to the publisher, Butch Cooper, for his patience, encouragement, and support. His personal belief in us and in the need to educate athletes and those who work with them about the insidious threat of performance-enhancing drug use made this project possible. Many physicians and scientists have contributed to our knowledge base regarding the origins, extent, and ramifications of this problem, only a few of who have been mentioned. No author in this field can fail to acknowledge the superb and voluminous contributions of Dr. Charles D. Kochakian in particular. Much gratitude is also due to the many athletes who, over the past 20 years, have described not only the appearance- and performance-enhancing effects of these drugs, but their effects on very intimate and personal aspects of their attitudes and life histories as well. A number of organizations should be commended for the steps they have taken to address this problem, including the American College of Sports Medicine and the National Strength and Conditioning Association. The efforts of the National Institute on Drug Abuse reflect a new level of awareness and commitment on the part of health professionals within the federal government to develop a consensus approach to the medical and social issues involved. Special thanks are also due to Dr. John Baenziger of the Drug Identification Laboratory at the Indiana University School of Medicine and to Don

Leggett and Dennis Degan of the U.S. Food and Drug Administration for their interest, and the information and photographs they graciously provided. Thanks also to Craig Gosling and Tex McArthur of the Indiana University School of Medicine Medical Illustration Department for their expert assistance with the photography.

James E. Wright, Ph.D.

First, I would like to thank George D. Lundberg, M.D., editor of the *Journal of the American Medical Association*; Phil Gunby, director of the division of JAMA Medical News and Perspectives and Humanities; and Richard H. Strauss, M.D., editor-in-chief of *The Physician and Sportsmedicine* for encouraging my interest in the field of drugs and sports and making it possible for me to pursue that interest and write about it, and to Don H. Catlin, M.D., director of the Paul Ziffren Olympic Analytical Facility at UCLA, for helping me develop a basic core of knowledge and for remaining one of my most trusted and respected sources.

Second, I would like to thank Charles Yesalis, Sc.D., for reading this manuscript in draft form, and Gary Wadler, M.D., and Brian Hainline, M.D., for their encouragement. Last, I would like to acknowledge the help of all those who have graciously given their time for interviews and who have made helpful suggestions over the years. Although that group now is too large to list individually, their contributions are significant.

Virginia S. Cowart

CONTENTS

1

SETTING THE SCENE

Each spring, some variation of the following scene is played out in high schools across the nation:

Coach: *Thanks for all your hard work, Jack. Keep it up this summer so you'll be in shape for fall. We'll be depending on you then, but champions are made in the off season, you know.*

Jack: *Got any suggestions, Coach? You know I want to put it all together next year. I'm really hoping for a college scholarship.*

Coach: *Well for a start, you need to gain about 20 pounds to be at a good playing weight. What's your bench press? About 220? Well, you need to get your bench press up as much as possible. And don't forget your squats and power cleans. With your talent, all you need to be a real standout is to grow some, get stronger and heavier, and keep your speed. Good luck.*

Next fall Jack returns bigger, stronger, more aggressive, and definitely college scholarship material. Coach is pleased to see that Jack took his advice. He likes Jack's attitude and work ethic, that he was willing to work so hard to help the team. Coach may never even so much as suspect that Jack resorted to drug use to achieve his gains in bulk and strength and, if he ever does suspect it, he may turn a blind eye to the evidence.

The evidence, both anecdotal and from surveys, suggests that many Jacks not only are working hard and taking various food and amino acid supplements. They also are using anabolic steroids or human growth hormone, or other performance-enhancing drugs and techniques such as blood doping to improve their athletic performance. They may be seasoned drug users by the time they graduate from high school.

Once drugs of elite athletes competing at the world-class level, anabolic steroids are now available to and being used by younger athletes and some teens who are not involved in competitive sports. Moreover, they are sometimes used with the tacit or expressed consent of their families and coaches. One San Diego school administrator said this type of drug use "is part of the whole yuppie thing, striving for success."

Striving for success may be a powerful reason for using anabolic steroids. Another may be that physical role models for young men and women are so extreme that few can meet them naturally. Just as anorexia nervosa is a body image disorder, anabolic steroid use may represent another facet of a body image distortion.

Initially, the use of anabolic steroids was confined to people who were competing at a high level and striving to gain even a small competitive edge. The question of which country's athletes were the first to take the field with steroids in their systems is debatable. The Americans have always said the honor belongs to the Russians, dating to the 1954 world weight lifting championships in Vienna. However, a British report claims that an American hammer thrower used steroids earlier than 1954.

Once drugs of elite athletes competing at the world-class level, anabolic steroids are now available to and being used by younger athletes and some teens who are not involved in competitive sports.

No matter which country was first, it didn't take long before steroids were commonplace. By 1956, their use was so pervasive that Olympian Olga Fikotova Connally said: "There is no way in the world a woman nowadays in the throwing events, at least the shot put and the discus, can break the record unless she is on steroids. These awful drugs have changed the complexion of track and field."

Nearly 35 years later, steroids are still an issue at the elite competitive level, but we have added a pool of much younger drug users, perhaps as many as 500,000.

Despite recent widespread publicity about anabolic steroids, recognition of steroid use by coaches, trainers, and parents appears to be lagging. For instance, a 1987-1988 survey of high school football coaches in Michigan showed that, while most coaches thought steroid use was inappropriate, **OVERALL, THEY DID NOT FEEL THE USE OF STEROIDS WAS A PROBLEM WITH HIGH SCHOOL FOOTBALL PLAYERS.** The emphasis here is ours but it is not misplaced. Until this problem is fully recognized, steps to correct it cannot be taken.

Here is a true story about one young "Jack" who began weight training to improve his size and strength for football. When he was 15 years old, Jack was 5 feet, 10 inches tall and weighed 175 pounds. After less than two months of weight training, he could bench press 225 pounds in strict form. His time for the 40-yard dash was 4.6 seconds. Jack's football career flourished.

While visiting relatives on the West Coast during the Christmas break of his senior year in high school, Jack dropped by a local gym where some of the regulars told him he could double or triple his muscle and strength gains simply by using anabolic drugs — specifically Dianabol — for six to eight weeks two or three times a year. Acne was the only possible side effect, they said, adding that it would disappear once he was off the drug. Jack didn't smoke and never abused alcohol, and he was reluctant to use steroids, especially after he talked with his family physician about them. However, he changed his mind after speaking with athletes at several colleges that were recruiting him to play football. Steroids were the ticket to success, they told him.

His family physician refused to prescribe steroids but Jack managed to obtain a 100-tablet bottle of 5 mg Dianabol for $30 from a weight lifter at his local gym. He went on a program that included a four-day-a-week combination power lifting/body building routine and a high protein, high carbohydrate, low fat diet of up to 6,000 calories a day. He also took 15 mg of Dianabol a day. Within five weeks, Jack's weight went from 210 to 222 pounds and his power lifting total went up 100 pounds.

Despite recent widespread publicity about anabolic steroids, recognition of steroid use by coaches, trainers, and parents appears to be lagging.

Jack began trying to locate more steroids, and this time purchased 200 tablets from another black market source. He took 15 mg a day for two weeks, then increased his daily dosage by 5 mg each week until the fifth week when he was consuming 30 mg of Dianabol a day. In the sixth, seventh, and eighth weeks of his drug cycle, he used 20, 10, and 5 mg Dianabol each day respectively, and he increased his body weight by another 11 pounds and his lifting total by 75 pounds. He noticed only a few side effects, mild acne on his face and shoulders, and a slight bloating of his face. In just three and a half months, Jack gained over 20 pounds and increased his bench press, squat, and deadlift total by 175 pounds. After seeing Jack's progress, close to a third of his high school team began using steroids that summer.

What hasn't been said yet about this story is that it happened in 1981 when steroids were neither as plentiful nor as well publicized as they are today.

In 1989, a Chicago high school football player told a reporter from the *Chicago Sun-Times* newspaper that he had injected steroids in his high school locker room in front of teammates.

"Everybody on the team knew what I was doing," he said. "They looked, but they didn't say anything. I think one coach knew, but he didn't want to say anything. Maybe he was afraid."

This young man started on steroids after he saw that a fellow student who used them as a freshman made the varsity team his sophomore year. He was able to purchase his illegal steroids easily, through his friend or at a private gym.

Young athletes seldom have to trouble themselves much to find a supplier.

Young athletes seldom have to trouble themselves much to find a supplier. When a Tampa radio station featured a call-in program on anabolic steroids late in 1989, one young man described how a schoolmate had invited him to his house and shown him a dresser drawer full of both oral and injectable steroids. Several other callers confirmed that obtaining steroids is almost as easy as buying aspirin at the drugstore (Figure 1-1).

A survey of high schools published in the *Journal of the American Medical Association* in 1988 showed that nearly 7 percent of the respondents had used at least one cycle of anabolic steroids by the time they were seniors. William Buckley, Ph.D., and Charles Yesalis, Sc.D., of Pennsylvania State University, and their colleagues asked 12th grade males in 46 private and public schools repre-

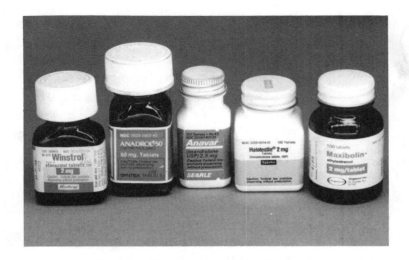

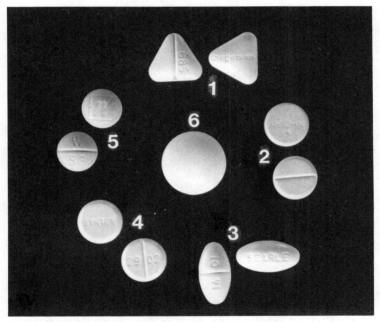

FIGURE 1-1. (Top) Five bottles of commonly used oral anabolic steroids. (Bottom) Five tablets (magnified 2.5 times) of commonly used oral steroids: 1 - ethylestrenol, 2 mg.; 2 - fluoxymesterone, 2 mg.; 3 - oxandrolone, 2.5 mg.; 4 - oxymetholone, 50 mg.; 5 - stanozolol, 2 mg.; and 6 - 325 mg. aspirin tablet displayed for size comparison.

senting a cross section of U.S. schools about steroids. About 40 percent of the users began before they were 16 years old, and 38 percent had used injectable forms of the drugs. Moreover, about 40 percent of the users admitted having been on five or more cycles (periods of use from six to 12 weeks in length) and they indicated they were unwilling to discontinue their use of steroids even in the face of possible health consequences.

...about 40 percent of the users...indicated they were unwilling to discontinue their use of steroids even in the face of possible health consequences.

In testimony before the House Subcommittee on Crime, Dr. Yesalis said if the study findings are extrapolated to the entire U.S. population, that means something like 250,000 adolescents have used anabolic steroids. The total number of anabolic steroids users in the United States is now estimated to be more than a million, Dr. Yesalis testified. That includes athletes, trainers, police, firefighters, military personnel, health club employes, and other people — mostly adolescents — who want to perform as well as possible as quickly as possible, and in some instances, with as little effort as possible.

Dr. Yesalis noted that there have been almost no studies to determine the actual prevalence of steroid use and those that have been done have been on athletes.

"It has been hypothesized, but not documented," he continued, "that the elite athletic population may be the smallest — but most visible

— user group and that a much larger user group exists comprised of lower level amateur and recreational individuals with perhaps other reasons for use."

Documenting the Problem

Because so little information is available on actual steroid use by adolescents, a Loyola University (Chicago) sociologist surveyed 2,113 students — both athletes and non-athletes — at another Chicago high school to see what information might emerge from a one-school study. Ninety-four students — 67 males and 27 females — admitted taking steroids. This is an overall incidence of 4.4 percent, a little lower than what Dr. Buckley and Dr. Yesalis estimated but a normal variance for only one school. (At the other end of the spectrum was an Arkansas high school study that showed 11 percent steroid use.) The dimensions of the steroid problem can be seen more clearly by the fact that 332 of the Chicago students (15.7 percent) reported that they knew someone who used steroids, and 732 students (34.6 percent) stated it would be easy to obtain steroids if they wanted them.

The need to document the extent of steroid use in athletics was emphasized at the 1989 American College of Sports Medicine meeting in Baltimore, Maryland, by Douglas B. McKeag, M.D., associate professor of family practice at Michigan State University. Dr. McKeag was an investigator for the 1984 and 1988 National Collegiate Athletic Association (NCAA) drug use and abuse surveys, and for the Michigan State University high school steroid survey of coaches.

In his summary, Dr. McKeag said bluntly, "Anabolic-androgenic steroids may constitute the single most significant threat to the integrity of sports in this country and drug use and abuse certainly constitutes the most significant threat to the future of sport. Intervention of some sort must occur for resolution of this problem."

"Anabolic-androgenic steroids may constitute the single most significant threat to the integrity of sports in this country..."

The NCAA survey data he presented at that meeting shows that anabolic steroid use has increased and that it is higher among high school students than it is among college students. Whereas 7 percent of high school athletes reported using anabolic steroids, only 5 percent of college athletes admitted to their use.

James Swenson, Jr., M.D., an assistant professor of orthopedics at the University of Rochester, surveyed Michigan high school football coaches in 1987-88, and found that most believed they would be able to detect steroid use among their athletes, but that they had less confidence in the ability of other coaches to do the same. This suggests the existence of the "blind eye" problem in coaching. Most coaches think highly of their teams and their reaction often is, "I know this kid and he couldn't be a drug user." Although this attitude may be more common when drugs are taken for performance enhancement, this disbelief or denial syndrome also happens with recreational drug use. When basketball star Len Bias died of a cocaine overdose, Maryland coach Lefty Driesell said, "I swear on my life, I hope to die if this kid ever used drugs before." Bias' old playground coach was so certain Bias didn't use drugs that he said, "I would have been willing to bet my whole house and my car."

Another significant finding from the Michigan coaches survey was that although most coaches characterized themselves as somewhat informed, many had several misconceptions about steroids.

The coaches agreed that education is the most important and effective part of controlling steroids, and they favored educational approaches combined with less severe penalties for athletes who were caught using anabolic steroids. At present, penalties for steroid use vary from college to college. Most require offenders to get counseling. Many high schools have no formal steroid policies.

At present, penalties for steroid use vary from college to college. Most require offenders to get counseling. Many high schools have no formal steroid policies.

Richard H. Strauss, M.D., editor-in-chief of *The Physician and Sportsmedicine*, says the traditional techniques that have been employed to control drug use are controlling the supply, education, and testing. Dr. Strauss, who is an associate professor of preventive medicine and internal medicine at Ohio State University, said that efforts to control the supply have not worked, and that both education and testing have been only partially effective.

Although everybody agrees on the need for more education about steroids, it also seems clear that just any "education program" won't do. Education could have a paradoxical effect on drug use, according to a report from Oregon.

In 1987, a group of medical students at the Oregon Health Sciences University, Portland, made three types of one-time interventions with local high school football teams. One group heard a lecture complete with slides, and were also given a handout summarizing the medical evidence on the dangers of steroids. Another group received the handout but did not hear a lecture. The third group served as a control.

To the dismay of the medical students, all three groups became more interested in steroids and all had an increase in the number of high school athletes who would consider using anabolic steroids to help obtain a college scholarship, or who would use them even if it caused a 50 percent risk of dying within 20 to 30 years.

The group repeated the experiment in 1988, except that they placed more stress on the dangers of steroid use. The results were virtually the same. Because of this, the Oregon group now believes that a one-time intervention is probably not effective. "What may be more important if you really want to change attitudes about steroids is to begin earlier and involve trainers, coaches, and parents," said one of the young physicians.

Doctors Not Heeded

A complicating factor for educational programs is that many youngsters are taking these very powerful sex hormones — that cause profound derangements of body chemistry and as yet unknown effects on behavior — with no medical control or monitoring. A serious communications problem exists between the medical community and most steroid users.

For some years, most doctors told athletes that steroids didn't work. Athletes simply stopped listening to them and looked to other sources for information. This sets a dangerous precedent in that steroid users are pursuing a course of action that carries a definite risk to health without the support of society's traditional caregivers. Users also may delay seeking medical treatment for steroid-related conditions.

The evolution of this communications gap can be traced back more than two decades to the first research that involved giving steroids to healthy people. When physicians recognized that anabolic steroids were being used to enhance sports performance, studies were undertaken to see if the claims that were being made by athletes could be confirmed scientifically. However, the first 25 scientific studies on steroids were divided on the question of effectiveness, with about half concluding that there were no beneficial effects on performance.

There were reasons why this was so. Some early studies contained flaws in the research design. The most common mistake was using untrained subjects, such as physical education students. We know now that the greatest gains with steroids occur in subjects who are experienced in strength training. Other design problems were with the length of study, caloric intake of subjects, and the drug dosages given.

When physicians read these results of the first studies, many became skeptical that steroids could provide anything more than a placebo effect — a phenomenon in which extremely positive results are gained when someone is given a totally inert substance that looks, smells, and tastes like a real drug. Moreover, there have been studies in which weight lifters made as much progress on placebos (often called "sugar pills") as they did on steroids, provided they were told and actually believed that the pills were steroids.

A serious communications problem exists between the medical community and most steroid users.

However, in other studies, 100 percent of the test subjects who were experienced in weight training and in the use and effects of steroids knew when they were on the drug, which raises the possibility that a double blind study may not be possible. (A double-blind study is one in which neither researcher nor test subjects know at the time a drug is given whether it is real or a placebo. This prevents bias from being introduced by the researcher.) Many people also fail to realize that just because the placebo effect does work does not mean that steroids don't. An athlete could benefit from both.

While scientists were doing their experiments, so were athletes. Using themselves as guinea pigs, many athletes were pleased to discover that steroids enabled them to lift heavier weights; work longer; run, bike, or swim faster; or throw farther.

Sports medicine experts and societies have acknowledged that they were wrong, but the breach between physicians and athletes has not been healed. Moreover, there are doctors who still insist that steroids do not help athletes enhance sports performance.

Looking at the Literature

During the time of noncommunication and mistrust between athletes and the scientific community, an underground literature sprang up to serve drug using athletes. Many users rely heavily on this underground steroid literature that often looks and sounds as scientific as any medical journal. The exaggerated drug claims that characterize this literature led one Canadian drug expert to say he enjoys reading it for entertainment.

Of the various publications for steroid users, the best known is probably *The Underground Steroid Handbook* which sold several thousand copies in a two-week period when it was recently updated. In fairness, it must be said that this publication does advise against children and teenagers taking steroids. It also tells readers to get a physical before they start using the drugs. However, on the down side, it states that the more steroids users take, the more they will grow, thus promoting heavier use and increasing the likelihood of adverse health effects.

Another monthly underground publication for steroid users, from Canada, evaluates various products as part of its "service" to readers. Following is a portion of its review of Testosterone Cypionate:

"Let me start out by saying that this drug is probably responsible for more muscle growth and more world power lifting records than any other injectable steroid ever. It has been the backbone for 80 pounds of muscle I've put on over the past three years. It is very androgenic and in turn very, very anabolic. It promotes muscle growth and tendon strength through protein synthesis. Its glycogen loading capabilities are unmatched by any other steroid available. Testosterone Cypionate is an excellent drug to aid in recuperation from heavy and intense workouts. It enables you to train harder and maintain a higher degree of recuperation ability than would normally be possible."

A naive reader might assume that these data are entirely factual. Readers who lack critical thinking skills seldom ask themselves about the quality of the research or whether it was conducted in line with generally accepted scientific practice. We don't know if the results reported here can be replicated by other researchers. Seldom in the underground literature are we told who is making the statements, what their qualifications are, and what evidence supports their claims. Unfortunately, most young athletes, and many older ones, not only are naive readers, but are not likely to turn to sources that might give them negative information they don't want.

Research Support Lags

It is true that when steroids first became a fact of life in the athletic community, some elite athletes worked out patterns of use and dosage levels that allowed them to achieve satisfactory results, but these individual experiments cannot be extrapolated to the population at large. Moreover, we still don't know whether some of these individuals will experience adverse affects later in life.

How the body reacts to anabolic steroids is affected by age, weight, genetic potential, diet, previous training and present conditioning programs. It is a very individualized proposition.

Reputable investigators are still doing steroid research, but they are forbidden by ethical and legal constraints to give volunteers the megadose amounts now being taken by some users. Sometimes they observe volunteer athletes who are self-administering steroids. Dr. Strauss has continued doing steroid research, and he likens it to doing astronomy.

Readers who lack critical thinking skills seldom ask themselves about the quality of the research or whether it was conducted in line with generally accepted scientific practice.

"We are looking at a population taking anabolic steroids in whatever way they wish, and studying those effects in a relatively haphazard way, like making observations of what is happening in another world," he says.

Sadly, financial support for scientific studies has not been forthcoming and Dr. Strauss comments: "A few of us have done studies, but it was basically unfunded research, accomplished by using volunteer, unpaid participation."

The result of this, he says, and other researchers agree, is that the potential problems have not been clearly identified in the user group. We know some of the short-term health effects, but we understand very little about the effects of multiple drugs in very high doses, which are sometimes taken for lengthy periods. An even more ominous fact: the long-term effects have not been studied, documented, and tested by the scientific community. The information is urgently needed if we are to encourage present users to stop taking anabolic steroids, and to convince young athletes they should never start.

2

STEROIDS AND HOW THEY WORK

Although many young men want to believe that anabolic steroids are wonder drugs, they are actually nothing other than synthetic male sex hormones — androgens. Naturally occurring androgens are the substances that are responsible for the transformation from boy to man, a process that occurs in every normal boy around the age of 13 or 14. However, long before hormones were ever identified as a class, observers already suspected that the development of male characteristics — including strength and power — was regulated in some way by the testes.

They had evidence to support this belief, both from commonplace observations and from scientific experimentation. Eunuchs were commonplace in the ancient world where it was an accepted practice to castrate some males, and their limited muscular development was well known. One of the earliest experiments to unlock the secrets of male/female differences occurred in 1771 in Scotland when John Hunter transplanted testes from a rooster to a hen and confirmed his theory that the hen would become more like a rooster. The very first steroid user might have been a doctor named Brown-Sequard who at age 72 administered a crude extract made from testes to himself in 1889. He reported a marked increase in strength, vitality, mental capacity, and digestive function, but could produce no scientific proof to back his claim.

A longing to be stronger and more powerful seems to be basic to the male mentality. To become another Atlas, or Hercules, or Sampson remains an ideal. We want our male heroes to have broad shoulders, muscular arms, narrow waists, and flat stomachs. They must be physically powerful, dominating, unyielding, and victorious.

That type of universal desire does not appear to be common to women, although female athletes want to develop enough strength and power to compete successfully in their sports. Yet, we do not want our heroines to look like our heroes. Women who have used anabolic steroids in a quest for strength and power often become so masculine in appearance that their gender needs to be confirmed for observers. Whether they have wished to become androgynous is open to question. The motivations for such drastic changes in appearance are complex and poorly understood, but they appear to be influenced by changes in culture and in the status of women in society.

Working out with weights or performing hard physical labor were the traditional paths to looking good physically for generations of adolescents and young adults until chemistry offered them a way to succeed beyond their wildest dreams. This is not to say that scientists were actually looking for a way to create a master race. Rather, the first scientific observations that confirmed the tissue-building effects of testicular hormones came about unexpectedly as a byproduct of scientific curiosity about energy metabolism.

A longing to be stronger or more powerful seems to be basic to the male mentality. To become another Atlas, or Hercules, or Sampson remains an ideal.

In 1935, after researchers identified testosterone as the masculinizing hormone that occurs naturally in the body, scientific interest soared. A young graduate research assistant at the University of Rochester produced one of the first clear demonstrations of the physical effects of a product of the testes. Charles D. Kochakian, Ph.D., reported a slight increase in energy metabolism accompanied by a dramatic reduction in nitrogen excretion in the urine of castrated dogs who had been given a potent androgen extract from human male urine. (Since nitrogen is the principal unique element in protein, the reduced excretion was first assumed and later proven to represent an increased formation of new body tissues — an anabolic effect.)

Dr. Kochakian conducted many of the pioneering studies on the anabolic and other effects of both natural and synthetic steroids on various body tissues and organs. However, Dr. Kochakian (now an emeritus professor at the University of Alabama Medical School in Birmingham) contends, along with other experts, that all new synthetic "anabolic" steroids should be called anabolic-androgenic steroids for the sake of accuracy. The reason: the tissue-building (anabolic) and virilizing (androgenic) effects of the new synthetic steroids cannot be completely separated.

Hormonal Control

The chemical action of synthetic anabolic steroids manufactured in a laboratory is similar to that of the naturally occurring male sex hormones. Hormones themselves are a class of powerful compounds produced by the endocrine glands. They are largely responsible for coordinating the chemical reactions in all the cells of the body.

An adult human has about 60 trillion cells in his body. Cells come in various sizes and shapes and are usually grouped into tissues (like muscle) that perform specialized functions (like contractions). The potential for cell growth is determined by the genetic material within it — the DNA — but cell growth cannot occur unless the environment is favorable. To grow, cells must have the appropriate quantity and quality of nutrients and the proper amounts of a variety of hormones.

We can think of hormones as the body's regulatory agency. (The word hormone was first used around the turn of the century by a British physiologist, and it comes from a Greek word meaning "setting in motion" or "arousing to activity.") Growth, metabolic rate, and blood chemistry are all controlled by hormones, which exert their effects in at least three ways:

- Hormones may exert a direct effect on intracellular enzyme systems to speed up or slow down certain reaction rates.

- Hormones may alter the supply of raw materials within cells by altering the permeability of the membranes surrounding the cells so that nutrients can pass into or out of them more or less easily.

- Hormones may activate or suppress particular genes so that the production of various substances is increased or decreased.

What we call a normal healthy physiological state is maintained only because of the delicate balance of hormones within the body, controlled by two "master" endocrine organs, the hypothalamus and the pituitary. Both of these master organs are located at the base of the brain (Figure 2-1), and they operate in a feedback loop like a thermostat. Both the hypothalamus and the pituitary secrete

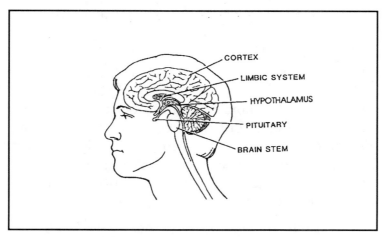

FIGURE 2-1. The two "master" endocrine organs, the hypothalamus and the pituitary, control the delicate balance of hormones within the body.

hormones that enter the circulation and stimulate production and release of other hormones to produce direct effects on organs. When the appropriate levels are reached, the amounts of hormone in circulation influence the master glands so that production levels are maintained within "normal" ranges.

Chemical analysis reveals that some hormones, including those manufactured by the pituitary, thyroid gland, and pancreas, are proteins. Other hormones, including those produced by the adrenal cortex, ovaries, and testes, are special types of lipids called steroids after a Greek word meaning "solid" or "firm." More than 500 different steroids have been identified in the human body. Cholesterol is the raw material of all the naturally occurring androgens and estrogens (female sex hormones).

Very little testosterone is stored in the testes of a normal adult male, so production must be more or less continuous. The average rate of testosterone production in a healthy young male is about 6 milligrams a day. The principal storage department for naturally produced androgens is the blood, where 98 percent or more of the body's testosterone is temporarily stored bound to proteins (albumin and globulin) circulating in the blood. The supply tends to remain relatively constant because the rate of testosterone production is controlled by another hormone, the luteinizing hormone (LH), which comes from the pituitary gland.

Women and young boys normally have only low concentrations of testosterone in their bodies, produced mainly by the adrenal glands. However, in adult males, only minute quantities of the testosterone supply is produced by the adrenal glands. Most of the testosterone in adult males is produced by special cells (Leydig cells) in the testes.

When young boys reach the age of puberty, their testes begin a sudden and sustained surge in testosterone production that peaks and levels off at about age 16 or 17. Even now, the events that cause this major hormonal change to occur are not completely understood. However, the results of a substantial increase in testosterone production are very apparent. Young men develop deeper voices, facial and body hair, enlargement and development of the genitals, awakening of sexual interest, and stronger, more powerful physiques.

Although the body's own androgenic-anabolic hormones play a role in growth and development, there are actually several other hormones that specifically influence growth, including growth hormone, thyroxin, insulin, and estrogens. A lack or deficiency in production of any of these hormones can upset the normal physiological state, sometimes with disastrous effects. For example, someone whose pituitary does not produce growth hormone is destined to be a dwarf unless he is treated with synthetic growth hormone.

What Are Steroids?

At the elementary chemical level, all steroids have the same basic four-ring carbon skeleton (Figure 2-2). Naturally occurring steroids differ in the number of carbon atoms attached to the number 17 carbon atom in the skeleton, and in the manner in which hydrogen (H), oxygen (O), and hydroxyl (OH) groups are attached to the carbon atoms.

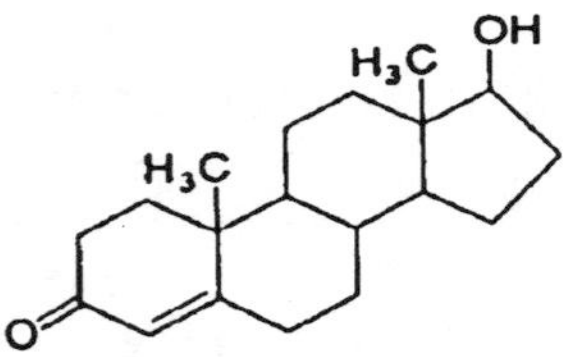

FIGURE 2-2. The chemical structure of testosterone.

The basic difference between naturally occurring androgens and the synthetic anabolic-androgenic steroids are that the chemical structure of the latter have been manipulated to enhance the anabolic (or tissue-building) characteristics of the natural hormone and to minimize the androgenic (or virilizing) characteristics. The various manipulations of chemical structure produce a number of different types of anabolic steroids (Tables 2-1 and 2-2), but all of them resemble the principal male sex hormone, testosterone. Their chemical structure also has been altered to prolong the lifespan of the steroid in the body. The idea was to promote the tissue-building effects at dose levels that minimize the occurrences of masculinizing effects. However, all experts agree that the tissue-building and virilizing characteristics cannot be completely separated. According to Dr. Kochakian, the anabolic and androgenic activities are distinguished primarily for classification purposes and not because of properties inherent in the steroids themselves.

How Steroids Work

If someone swallowed plain testosterone, it would have virtually no effect because the liver would rapidly break it down and inactivate it through metabolism. Injection of testosterone is

Table 2-1. *Oral Anabolic Steroids - Reference List*

The following list includes some examples of generic and trade names of oral anabolic steroids. This list was compiled from the 29th Edition of *MARTINDALE The Extra Pharmacopeia,* London: The Pharmaceutical Press, 1989. For a more comprehensive list, including oral steroids available some years ago, consult the text by Kochakian listed in the references.

Generic Name	Trade Name(s)
Calusterone:	Methosarb
Danazol:	Danocrine, Danol, Cyclomen, Danatrol, Danobrin, Ladogar, Winobanin
Ethylestrenol:	Maxibolin, Orabolin, Orgabolin
Fluoxymesterone:	Android-F, Halotestin, Oralsterone, Oratestin, Ora-Testryl, Ultandren
Furazabol:	Miotolon
Mebolazine:	Roxilon
Mesterolone:	Mestoranum, Proviron
Methandriol:	Sinesex, Stenediol, Troformone
Methandrostenolone/Methandienone:	
	Andoredan, Danabol, Dianabol, Encephan, Lanabolin, Metabolina, Metanabol, Metastenol, Nerobol, Perbolin, Metaboline (a multi-ingredient preparation that also contains methandrostenolone)
Methenolone (acetate):	
	Primobolan
Methyltestosterone:	Androyd, Glosso-Sterandryl, Mesteron, Metandren, Neo-Hombreol, Neohombreol-M, Orchisterone, Oreton, Methyl, Perandren, Primotest, Testin, Testomet, Testoviron, Testovis, Testred, Virilon, Virormone-Oral
Mibolerone:	Cheque Drops
Norethandrolone:	Nilevar
Oxandrolone:	Anavar, Antitriol, Lonavar
Oxymesterone:	Anamidol, Balnimax, Oranabol, Oranabol 10
Oxymetholone:	Anapolon-50, Anadrol 50, Adroyd, Anadroyd, Anasteron, Anasteronal, Nastenon, Oxitosona-50, Pardroyd, Plenastril, Synasteron, Zenalosyn
Quinbolone:	Anabolicum Vister
Stanozolol:	Winstrol, Stromba
Testosterone undecanoate:	
	Restandol

Table 2-2. *Injectable Anabolic Steroids - Reference List*

The following list includes some examples of generic and trade names of injectable anabolic steroids. This list was compiled from the 29th Edition of *MARTINDALE: The Extra Pharmacopeia,* London: The Pharmaceutical Press, 1989. For a more comprehensive list, including injectable steroids available some years ago, consult the text by Kochakian listed in the references.

Generic Name   **Trade Name(s)**
Boldenone Undecylenate:
                          Equipose, Vebonal
Dromostanolone (Drostanolone) propionate:
                          Masteril, Masteron, Metormon, Permastril, Drolban
Formebolone: Esiclene, Hubernol
Furazabol: Miotolone
Methandrostenolone: Dianabol
Methenolone esters (acetate and enanthate):
                          Primobolan, Primobolan Depot, Primobolan S,
                          Primonabol
Nandrolone esters (primarily the phen(yl) propionate and decanoate)
                          Anabolin LA-100, Androlone, Deca-Durabolin,
                          Durabolin, Hybolin Decanoate, Kabolin, Nandrolin,
                          Neo-Durabolic and many others
Oxabolone cypionate: Steranabol Depot, Steranabol Ritardo
Stanozolol: Winstrol-V, Anasyth, Stromba, Strombaject, Winstrol
Stenbolone acetate: Stenobolone
Testosterone (suspension, and various esters, primarily propionate, enan-
thate, and cypionate):
                          Andriol, Andronate, BayTestone, Delatestryl,
                          Depo-Testosterone, Jectatest-LA, Malogen LA,
                          Sterandryl, Sustanon, Testate, Testone LA,
                          Testostroval-PA, and many others, including
                          multi-ingredient preparations
Trenbolone acetate: Parabolan, Finajet, Finaplix

more effective, but metabolism still occurs very quickly. Chemical modifications have to be made to enable the body to use these drugs.

To prevent rapid breakdown by the liver, oral steroids are subjected to a process called alkylation (Figure 2-3), and injectable steroids are enhanced through a process known as esterification (Figure

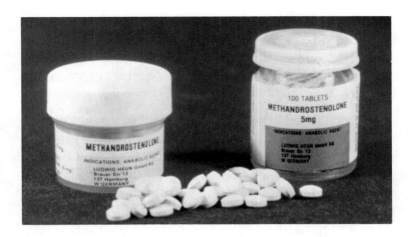

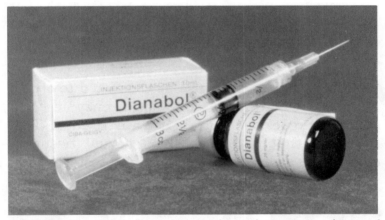

FIGURE 2-3. *(Top) The oral and most common form of methandrostenolone, an alkylated anabolic steroid. (Bottom) An injectable version of methandrostenolone available only in low dosage concentrations due to the limited oil solubility of such alkylated drugs. Used mostly in veterinary medicine, it was approved for human use in some countries. Oral methandrostenolone was for years the anabolic steroid most widely used by athletes attempting to add strength and muscle mass. Although no longer available through CIBA anywhere, generic equivalents are still available in some countries. Substances labeled Dianabol or methandrostenolone but which may contain none of this material are still sold on the black market in many places. The 1988 Anti-Drug Abuse Act reclassified methandrostenolone as a Schedule I drug, the same as heroin, meaning it has high abuse potential and no legitimate medical use.*

2-4). Esterified anabolic steroids are highly soluble in lipid and are stored in body fat. Because they are absorbed over a longer period of time, esterified anabolic steroids can be more easily detected by drug testing.

✳ Once inside the body, about 98 to 99 percent of steroids become attached, or bound to plasma proteins. Only the one percent or so that isn't bound is what gets taken up into the cells of the body. The free steroid enters a cell by simple diffusion. These free steroids may then bind directly to the receptors, as testosterone does in muscle tissue (Figure 2-5). Binding is a method of "unlocking" the cell response, which simply means that if protein synthesis is taking place, the cell's normal response will be altered by the presence of the testosterone.

Free steroids may also be converted to other, more active substances by special enzymes and chemical reactions within certain tissues. Testosterone that enters a cell of sexual tissue is changed to a chemical called dihydrotestosterone, which is responsible for its effects there. Tes-

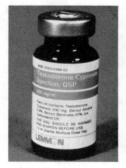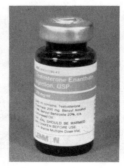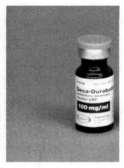

FIGURE 2-4. *These are samples of the most commonly used esterified anabolic steroids: (left) Testosterone cypionate; (center) Testosterone evanthate; and (right) Nandrolone decanoate.*

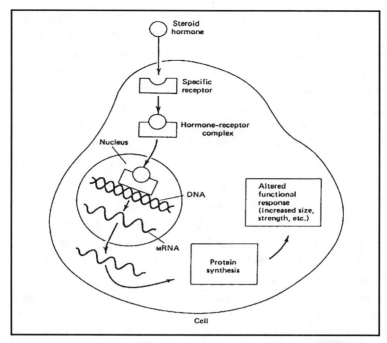

FIGURE 2-5. *This simplified model describes how steroid hormones affect cell growth. Steroid hormone enters the cell and binds to a receptor molecule. The bound hormone can then enter the nucleus and activate specific genes to produce proteins. These proteins in turn bring about the cellular changes triggered by the hormone.*

tosterone and some anabolic steroids can also be converted to estrogens within cells of the brain, liver, fat, and muscle, and cause the typical effects associated with these hormones.

By virtue of their specific chemical structure (which is totally different from any vitamin or amino acid), anabolic steroids are able to stimulate the genetic apparatus (DNA) within the cell nucleus. The DNA reacts to this stimulation by directing the production of specific new proteins.

It is very important to understand that the biological response that occurs is dependent on the location and number of the receptors. If the receptor is in muscle, there will be a tissue-building effect. If the receptor is in the brain, there may be noticeable psychological and possibly even behavioral effects. There are, incidentally, more receptors in "sexual" tissues than in muscle, which raises concern about the prospect of hypertrophy or cancer of the prostate gland.

If the body's receptors are already saturated with testosterone, no further tissue-building effects will occur with continued dosage. Normally, however, the steroid receptors in a man's muscle tissue are about half saturated by his own testosterone production. Training will increase the attraction of receptors for anabolic steroids. Training that increases muscle size also increases the number of receptors available to bind to anabolic hormones. Another key ingredient in the process is maintaining adequate nourishment for the developing muscle tissue. A steroid user must take in more calories, especially proteins and complex carbohydrates, to maximize the addition of mass and strength.

The receptors in the muscle tissue of women are not saturated with testosterone, so they tend to see immediate and striking changes when they use anabolic steroids. Besides increased muscular development, they often see other undesirable and sometimes permanent changes, such as body and facial hair, enlarged genitals, and deeper voices.

Boys who have not gone through puberty or who are just beginning the process will get striking changes also. They will develop bodies that look more mature, but there is a danger that the growth plates on the ends of their bones will close prematurely, causing them to be shorter than they otherwise would have been. There is growing concern that flooding a young adolescent with synthetic sex hormones may disrupt not only physical changes but also normal psychological and emotional maturation that occurs during adolescence.

Fooling Mother Nature

Not long after the first studies on hormonal manipulations, speculation began about possible uses for anabolic steroids. As early as 1939, European researcher Ove Boje foresaw the future by suggesting (in a report from the Health Organization of the League of Nations) that administration of sex hormones might theoretically improve athletic performance. His suggestion did not remain on the theoretical level for long. It appears that various forms of testosterone were used by body builders to increase muscle size and strength in the late 1940s, although the entry of steroids into international competition came later.

It wasn't until 1953 that researchers observed that a certain chemical modification of testosterone (removal of the 19th carbon atom) resulted in a compound that was able to induce tissue-building effects at dose levels that evoked only minimal androgenic activity (only about a third as much as testosterone). This compound, Norethandrolone (marketed in 1956 by Searle as Nilevar), was the first commercially available "anabolic steroid." A related version was esterified to enhance its solubility in oil and to prolong its release and duration of action, and it was introduced in 1959 as nandrolone phenylpropionate (marketed by Organon as Durabolin). Syntex released oxymetholone in 1960, Sterling-Winthrop provided stanozolol in 1962, and Searle introduced oxandrolone in 1964.

The receptors in the muscle tissue of women are not saturated with testosterone, so they tend to see immediate and striking changes when they use anabolic steroids.

CIBA Pharmaceuticals introduced methandrostenolone, also known as methandienone, (Dianabol) in 1958, and as reports of its effectiveness spread, it quickly became one of the most widely used anabolic steroids in the world. In 1981, the U.S. sales of this product were $1.5 million. CIBA withdrew Dianabol for human use in 1982, ostensibly because other medications were available to treat patients for whom the steroid had been prescribed. It continued to sell veterinary Dianabol until 1985, but a company spokesperson said Dianabol is no longer available anywhere in the world through CIBA. The 29th (1989) edition of *MARTINDALE The Extra Pharmacopeia*, however, lists methandrostenolone as available under a variety of trade names in numerous countries around the world. Counterfeit products continue to be available on the U.S. black market.

Steroids in Medicine

Most early thinking about how to use anabolic steroids was along traditional medical lines, such as the proposal in 1942 by Alan Kenyon, M.D., that they might be effective in treating some war casualties. Anabolic steroids do have legitimate medical uses, of course. The principal physiological basis for their clinical use is their stimulation of protein synthesis.

Physicians primarily prescribe steroids as replacement therapy for patients whose hormone production is low, for patients with certain types of anemias, and for those with a relatively rare inherited condition called angioneurotic edema. Steroids are sometimes prescribed for patients who are malnourished from disease or some other factor like advanced age. Steroids may be used to treat skeletal disorders because they stimulate formation of the protein matrix of bone and protect against agents that might interfere. Surgeons sometimes prescribe steroids to improve a patient's overall condition before operating or, as the Russians sometimes do, to promote wound healing afterward. They have been used to treat fibrocystic breast disease, female breast cancer, endometriosis, and osteoporosis. Some pediatric experts such as Alan Rogol, M.D., an endocrinologist at the University of Virginia, Charlottesville, have studied anabolic steroids as a potential way to stimulate growth in patients who are abnormally short or whose normal pubertal development is delayed.

In the 1970s, the World Health Organization (WHO) began studying synthetic testosterone as a possible male contraceptive. Male study subjects were given doses of 200 to 300 mg per week for up to 18 months. That project is ongoing at several locations throughout the world.

Before these options were open to physicians, researchers had to demonstrate the beneficial effects of anabolic steroids in animals. Much of the basic animal work used rats to demonstrate the effects of testosterone. Early research showed that one particular muscle of castrated male rats, the levator ani, became bigger and stronger when testosterone was administered. However, while the levator ani is a part of the male reproductive system, it is unique to male rodents. Although the animal studies with rats, and later with dogs, provided valuable information, we must note that conclusions from such studies may not be directly applicable to patients receiving steroids as medical therapy, much less to healthy young people.

Steroids are used routinely and legitimately in veterinary medicine (Figure 2-6). They are given to horses to enhance the rate of growth and muscle mass. Race horses usually begin training at about 13 months of age, which is comparable to a preadolescent age in a human. Steroids help horses endure the musculoskeletal stress of heavy-impact

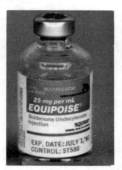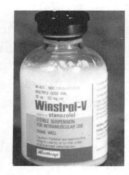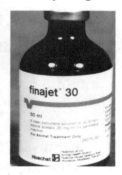

FIGURE 2-6. *The samples above are veterinary anabolic steroids often used by athletes but not approved as safe for use in humans by the U.S. Food and Drug Administration: (left) Bolderone undecylenate; (center) Stanozolol; and (right) Trenbolone acetate, which is not even approved for veterinary use in this country. Counterfeits of all these substances have been confiscated; some contained no active ingredients and others contained dangerous and even lethal substances. Penicillin, which can be fatal to allergic individuals, has been found in Winstrol-V.*

training. They gain more muscle mass and develop larger hearts.

Charting the Effects

During the two decades after testosterone was identified as the source of masculinization, investigators studied the effects on many of the body tissues and organs. They found that skeletal muscles are very sensitive to testosterone, a sensitivity that can be demonstrated by the decrease in muscle mass that follows castration. Also, the size of several organs, notably the kidney, heart, and liver, is affected by the level of circulating testosterone. Fat deposits under the skin and around the internal organs increase in the bodies of men who lack sufficient amounts of testosterone, and the number of red blood cells available for oxygen transport decreases. The beneficial effects of testosterone on the body are considered to be the "anabolic" or tissue-building effects. The "androgenic" or masculinizing effects include growth of the penis and accessory sex glands, increase in facial and body hair, deepening of the voice, increased oiliness of the skin, and enhancement of sexual interest.

Information from both animal and human studies on steroids can be summed up as follows:

- The most profound metabolic action of androgens is the formation and storage of tissue protein — or protein anabolism. Less nitrogen, phosphorus, potassium, calcium (and, at times, sodium and chloride) are lost. When androgen treatment is stopped, there usually is a temporary increase in nitrogen excretion and some loss (occasionally a great deal) of the weight gained.

- The effect on protein synthesis probably returns to normal levels after existing protein deficiencies have been overcome. The tissue-building effect, signaled by nitrogen retention, usually begins within two to three days after androgens are given. (Some steroids act quickly while others begin stimulation more slowly but have more prolonged effects.) In normal animals, nitrogen balance returns to normal after a few days but the "wearing off" effect occurs later in animals that are deficient in either natural androgen or protein.

- Androgenic hormones cause an increase in RNA in the nucleus of the cell and in protein-building enzymes at the basic level. The activities of other enzymes involved in energy metabolism also are increased.

- Muscles within the same body vary in response to androgen treatment. Muscles of the shoulder girdle area seem to be most affected in humans. However, other factors also affect muscle response, including age, sex, nutritional status, and training status. Some experts believe that steroids increase the blood transport network in muscle tissue. In any event, androgens do not necessarily confer a whole body, or universal effect.

- The accessory sex glands, and perhaps the kidney, accumulate protein before other tissues do.

- Androgens have not been conclusively shown to change the metabolic rate, but there may be a shift toward greater utilization of fat. A good deal of evidence suggests that steroids decrease visceral and total carcass body fat while increasing the protein and water content. Even so, the overall influence of steroids on fat tissue and fat metabolism is still unclear.

- Both protein and caloric intake must be adequate to get a maximum tissue-building effect of steroids. However, experiments on normal animals (not exercise trained) showed that simply increasing the protein content above 18 percent of the total calories in the diet did not improve nitrogen retention. The rate of protein synthesis is related to the intake of calories, and will not be maximal unless a surplus of calories is consumed.

- Excessive doses of androgen inhibit growth in young rats, an effect that is more apparent in normal male rats. Very large steroid dosages may result in a loss of protein (especially from the skin), probably from the reduction in appetite caused by the drug dosages, and a decrease in fat tissue so that there may be a weight loss. What the implications of these animal findings might have for young human steroid users is not known.

- Steroids appear to stimulate the formation of new bone tissues or the strengthening of the existing protein matrix in bone. Calcium retention begins slightly later than nitrogen retention, but it lasts longer and there isn't a rebound effect when steroids are discontinued.

- Wound healing appears to be accelerated. This has not been well studied in the U.S. but both the European and Russian medical literature contains reports of anabolic steroids being used for this purpose. Wound healing could be affected in a variety of ways. (It seems likely that some U.S. physicians who have prescribed anabolic steroids for athletes, particularly football players, have done so to counteract tissue damage or promote healing.)

Steroids in Sports

It is hard to sort out exactly what gains athletes make by using steroids since they commonly take mixtures of drugs and very large dosages. The effect of any one substance is difficult to determine.

A major point on which most scientists and some athletes agree is that anabolic steroids do not increase aerobic capacity, which is the rate at which the body can take in and use oxygen. An athlete can increase his ability to deliver oxygen to exercising muscles by training, but only up to a genetically preset maximum. Anabolic steroids can increase the volume of the blood, its oxygen-carrying capacity, and even heart size, but only one of 11 studies demonstrated consistent improvements in aerobic performance from steroid use. However, there could be an indirect effect, in that the anticatabolic effect of steroid use would permit an endurance athlete to train longer and harder, and the training itself might favorably affect aerobic capacity.

We also know that steroids have little effect by themselves. Someone not actively engaged in rigorous weight training and whose diet is normal will not experience any significant or lasting changes in muscle mass and strength with steroids, although there may be an effect on sexual behavior and mood. If a person believes that simply taking a pill or injection will make him "look good," he should be prepared for acne, hair loss, fluid retention, and disappointment.

The old theory that you have to tear down your muscles to build them up is, in a sense, true. Protein catabolism — a destructive process in which these chemical substances are broken down — is essential to growth. The more experienced an athlete is, and the longer and harder he or she trains, the more able that person is to do a catabolic exercise program. For this reason, the first change that beginning weight lifters notice is that strength comes before size. There is a motor learning phase that muscles must go through before they become bigger.

If a person believes that simply taking a pill or injection will make him "look good," he should be prepared for acne, hair loss, fluid retention, and disappointment.

Most of the first steroid users did not begin taking the drugs until they had reached a plateau in physical development, whereas many young users start taking steroids before they have developed much of their physical potential, and some begin using steroids when they first begin training.

Besides intensity of physical training and diet, other factors that play a role include heredity and the dosage of drug taken. Even if exercise and diet are adequate, not every steroid user will see strength gains greater than those that occur with training alone. Others will achieve only small gains — but small gains can be critically important in high level competition.

The role of intense weight training is confirmed by the scientific evidence. Referring again to the early studies on steroids, if they are divided into those that used weight-trained individuals and those that did not, it becomes apparent that the strongest effects will be observed in the trained subjects.

Even if exercise and diet are adequate,
not every steroid user will see strength gains
greater than those that occur with
training alone.

A pair of studies by a British team of researchers had enormous influence in changing the position of the scientific community on whether steroids affect sports performance. The double-blind studies were carried out at the University of Leeds, England, by a team under the leadership of G.R. Hervey, M.D. The first study used 11 untrained but athletic male physical education students who began by doing a two-week period of specified weight training. Then half the subjects received 100 mg methandrostenolone (Dianabol) a day for six weeks, while the other half received a placebo. At the end of the six-week drug cycle, all subjects stopped training for five weeks. They resumed training for one week before beginning a second six-week drug-taking cycle in which those who first received the drug now received the placebo and vice versa. No food supplements were given. The leg press was used as a measure of whether strength improved. As could be expected, performance in the training exercises improved significantly over both periods, but the strength gains in the steroid-taking group were no greater than those from training alone. Moreover, strength decreased rapidly when the drugs were stopped.

Next, Dr. Hervey repeated his 13-week experiment with seven experienced weight trainers. The second group of subjects were somewhat older and heavier than the first, but they took the same drug and dosages. The average weight gain during the six weeks of steroid use was 2.3 kilograms, mainly in lean muscle tissue. There were obvious increases in muscle size. Weight lifting performance and leg strength increased significantly more with steroid use than in the placebo group. The amounts of nitrogen and potassium in the bodies of the drug group increased significantly, disproportionately in fact to the amount of weight gained. These data confirmed the often dramatic weight and strength gains that had been reported anecdotally by athletes.

Another example of a well-controlled, double-blind study using non-weight trained subjects was published in 1965 by William Fowler, M.D., and his colleagues at the University of California at Los Angeles. Forty-seven healthy college students were divided into two experimental groups and two control groups. One experimental group received only the drug while the other drug group also followed an exercise program. One control group received only a placebo, and the other received the placebo and followed the specified exercise program. Both groups that exercised increased their aerobic work capacity, but there were no significant changes in body weight, muscle size, or skinfold thickness in any group. This is what we would expect, given our current state of knowledge about steroids.

A study that did use weight trained subjects was carried out at UCLA by V.R. Edgerton, Ph.D., and three colleagues. They followed and tested six competitive Olympic weight lifters while these athletes undertook a program of training and drug self-administration over a 12-week period. The lifters had between one and 12 years competitive experience. The drug dosages they took would be considered extremely low by today's standards.

Before, during, and after that period, the researchers measured body weight, fat, and a profile of 24 biochemical parameters in blood. A sample of tissue from the outer thigh was taken before and after the 12-week period so it could be evaluated for size and chemical changes. Strength also was measured periodically. The findings can be summarized by saying that all gained body weight and that body fat decreased. The biopsy results indicated that the individual fast twitch (Type II) muscle fibers (the ones that adapt to fast, high intensity anaerobic contractions) were larger in each subject after training and drug administration. There were significant changes in blood chemistry with regard to cholesterol, iron, total protein, and in an enzyme involved in lactic acid metabolism. However, few of these changes exceeded normal values. Although there were no control subjects, this study demonstrates the effectiveness of short-term, low-dose anabolic hormones in weight-trained individuals, something athletes have observed in gyms for 30 years. The lifter who took the highest drug dose was also the only one to take both oral and injected steroids, and he did not increase his lifts as much as four of the others did.

When a user ceases taking steroids, he can expect a significant loss of strength and size that may contribute to adverse mood effects, including depression. Loss of size and strength may not be as apparent in an adolescent user who is in a growth phase. However, there is evidence to support the view that users likely will lose some, and perhaps even a substantial proportion of their steroid-induced strength and body mass.

When a user ceases taking steroids, he can expect a significant loss of strength and size that may contribute to adverse mood effects, including depression.

One of the final questions that someone who is considering taking anabolic steroids must ask himself is: Is it worth it? Many elite athletes have concluded that the benefits do outweigh the risks. However, most research indicates that, without intensive strength training, the reverse is true. If the commitment to strength training is not strong, only modest, transitory gains may be experienced. And even where the training is intense and the commitment total, there are moral, legal, and health risks that argue overwhelmingly against the use of steroids.

3

HEALTH EFFECTS OF ANABOLIC STEROIDS

Many younger users of anabolic steroids prefer to skip right to the bottom line. Do steroids work? Will they kill me? If the answer to the first question is "Yes" and the answer to the second is "Probably not," that's all they want to hear.

Yet they need to hear more. There are health risks, known and unknown. Gymlore tends to dismiss reports of bad effects from anabolic steroids as scare talk aimed at frightening kids away from drugs that will make them bigger and stronger.

The truth is that, so far as we know right now, many of the short-term effects of steroids in males (acne, sterility, changes in blood fats, testicular shrinkage) are reversible. Acne, infertility, and blood fat changes are also reversible effects in women steroid users. However, some of the masculinizing effects, such as body hair growth, clitoral enlargement, and voice changes, are permanent.

Many experts believe, and we agree, that the three main unanswered questions about the potential health effects of steroids are:

- Do they cause psychological or physical dependence?

- Are they a gateway to other drug use?

- What hazards are associated with the fact that so many of the drugs available for sale are counterfeit and of unknown purity and potency?

Those are just the top of a long list of questions about steroids for which there are no answers yet. We don't know what the long-term effects on physical and mental health are, what the behavioral effects are and who is likely to experience them, whether long-term use of sex hormones may affect unborn children, and whether some adverse effects are related to dosage or the length of time drugs are taken. We don't know whether some anabolic steroids have more of a health risk than others. Are long-term steroid users at greater risk than those who took them only for short periods? Again, we don't know. We also don't know if younger steroid users have a greater risk of adverse effects. We don't know whether the risk is multiplied for users who take various combinations of hormones or other drugs.

Steroid users who have not experienced any adverse effects aren't yet in the clear because the lapse between associating cause and effect can sometimes be very long in medicine. AIDS is an example of a disease where there was a long interval (during which the infection spread) before the syndrome was recognized. Many people were unaware for years of their deadly peril. Yet another example is the hormonal time bomb that was launched when women took diethylstilbestrol (DES) in the 1950s to prevent miscarriage and unwittingly put their daughters at risk of uterine cancer and various other deformities. In March 1990, newspapers reported the death from this type of cancer of the 13-year-old granddaughter of a DES patient. Smoking is the most obvious example of a type of drug use that carries enormous delayed risks to health. Many young people still smoke, even though there are about 400,000 deaths a year from smoking- associated disease.

With anabolic steroids, we have not had enough time or a large enough group of identified older users to know whether significant health effects in later life will be seen.

Drug Sources

Before we talk about the dangers of the drugs themselves, we want to note that there is a risk to health simply from taking counterfeit drugs purchased on the black market. The Food and Drug Administration is as concerned about the health effects of counterfeit substances as it is about bona fide anabolic steroids, according to a spokesman. He had a bottle of counterfeit Dianabol that was seized in a raid and which actually contained 5 mg aspirin. Another drug expert has a bottle of "steroids" that actually contain nothing but caffeine, although it costs the purchaser much more than any caffeinated product.

According to John Bolton, an assistant attorney general: "Not only are we concerned with the risks associated with the unprescribed use of legitimate steroids (by adolescents), risks such as upsetting the hormonal balance and stunting growth, but of equal or greater concern is the unauthorized use of illegitimate steroids which have no FDA approval and are made under less than sanitary conditions. We think it's a very dangerous problem...You will see a lot more prosecutions."

The sources for obtaining steroids changed between 1985 and 1989, as indicated in Table 3-1. Obviously, it is more difficult today to get a physician to prescribe steroids for an athlete. That means that more drugs are being obtained on the black market. Estimates are that a third are counterfeit, a third are smuggled in from other countries, and a third are diverted from legitimate manufacturing sources, including those that make veterinary steroids. A veterinary journal recently reported that 90 percent of veterinary drugs supposed to be available only by prescription can be obtained without one. The counterfeit and smuggled drugs may pose substantial health risks be-

Table 3-1. *Sources for steroid users in 1985 and 1989.*

	1985	1989
Nonteam physicians	25%	10%
Team physicians	5%	0
Teammates	22%	49%
Friends/relatives	22%	29%
Coaches	5%	2%
Prof. scouts/agents	2%	4%
Other	22%	6%

Source: Report to the American College of Sports Medicine, June 1, 1989, "Drug Use and Abuse in Athletics."

cause they may be unsterile, or they ma
substances more harmful than the actu
they purport to be.

Behavioral Effects

Turning to the adverse health effects seen with anabolic steroid use, many experts are very concerned right now about the potential psychological and behavioral effects of taking steroids. These included drug dependence, depression, suicidal thoughts, and extremely aggressive behavior. Experts agree that there is strong evidence that some users do lose emotional control, and that we have no reliable way to predict who will have emotional or behavioral problems.

It is only fair to say up front that not everyone agrees that psychiatric effects may be a problem and, in fact, they were not demonstrated in earlier research studies. Some long-time steroid users have never suffered any emotional instability, or anything more than transient physical effects.

When steroid users discuss how their emotions are affected by anabolic steroids, many mention feelings of euphoria, well-being, and self-confidence. One speaker at a seminar on anabolic steroids sponsored by the National Institute of Drug Abuse commented that the "self confidence" cited may be more a lack of restraint than true self confidence. There are a number of cases now on record where lack of personal restraint by steroid users has led to legal restraint.

Psychiatrists Harrison G. Pope Jr., M.D., and David L. Katz, M.D., described several cases of homicide and near-homicide committed by anabolic steroid users. One apparently normal young man, with no symptoms of psychiatric disorder, rarely drank alcohol and had never used illicit drugs. He had no criminal record or past history of violent behavior. He worked as a prison security officer and had been happily married for several years. At age 27, the young man took up weight lifting, and at age 30 started on steroids, taking methandrostenolone (20 mg a day). During two of the six-week drug taking periods known as cycles, he combined somatotrophin and oxandrolone with the methandrostenolone. By the time he began his fifth six-week cycle, he had increased the dose to 30 mg of methandrostenolone a day, and added testosterone cypionate (300 mg a week) and methenolone (one injection of unknown dosage).

Experts agree that there is strong evidence that some users do lose emotional control, and that we have no reliable way to predict who will have emotional or behavioral problems.

Dr. Pope and Dr. Katz reported that his wife and coworkers noticed that the young man became markedly irritable and aggressive when he was on steroids, although in his opinion he was merely very self-confident. These mood changes were most noticeable at the higher drug doses. He became frankly emotionally disturbed during his fifth drug cycle and believed that the inmates at the prison were talking about him, and that his wife was plotting against him. He heard voices and had the sensation someone was touching him on the shoulder. His life spun out of control. After experiencing car trouble one day, he stopped at a local store to use the telephone and report he would be late to work. The woman at the store joked that

people from the prison used her phone so m\
should charge for it. The young man brooded
the remark, believing the woman had be
him. The next morning he drove back to the ____
and forced the woman into his car with no clear
motive, except to "scare" her. Although the subject
managed to drive off with the woman, she leaped
from the car when he was forced to stop for construction work after a short distance. As she fled,
the young man pulled his revolver and shot her in
the spine, leaving her a paraplegic. He was arrested and is now in prison. Although he suffered
a major depression after his arrest and withdrawal
from drugs, he has since returned to what Dr. Pope
and Dr. Katz believe is his normal personality.

Dr. Pope, who has an academic appointment
at Harvard University, and Dr. Katz, who is now
at Duke University, were the first to publish a
report detailing major psychiatric problems in
steroid users, although there have been anecdotal
reports for years, most often about the un-
restrained aggressiveness that goes by the name
"Roid Rage." In the Pope and Katz study, the 41
steroid users interviewed had a variety of
syndromes, including manic episodes, major
depression, delusions, and hallucinations.

A suicide brought to our attention recently
involved a teen-age youth who had previously in-
jured his knee in a motorcycle accident. His doctor
prescribed the anabolic steroids Anavar and Deca-
Durabolin for a three- to four-month trial to see if
they aided his rehabilitation. After watching
television one afternoon with a friend at whose
home he was staying, he went into his bedroom,
placed a shotgun in his mouth and pulled the

trigger. His friends said he had not displayed suicidal tendencies, and his mother believes that the steroids were responsible for his death.

If natural biological changes can cause such marked shifts of mood, how much more dramatic must they be in someone who is ingesting or injecting very high doses of male sex hormones?

More criminal cases in which the defendant is a steroid user are being reported. One of the first was an arson and burglary case involving a young man with a previously good record in the U.S. Navy who took up weight lifting and who eventually began taking steroids. After going through several cycles of heavy steroid use, he broke into houses and set several of them on fire. Yet another steroid case involved a young man who was so obsessed with bodybuilding that he took extremely high doses of steroids. At Ricky Wayne Boblett's trial in Virginia for attempting to kill his girlfriend — first by planting a bomb under her car and later by trying to hire a hit man — the defense claimed steroids were responsible for his dramatic mood swings between depression and aggression. Medical testimony was given to support this claim.

The fact that hormonal shifts can play havoc with emotions is a fact of life known by the parents of nearly any teen going through puberty or any woman going through menopause. Euphoria may accompany the large increase in sex hormones that occur during pregnancy. If natural biological changes can cause such marked shifts of mood, how much more dramatic must they be in someone who is ingesting or injecting very high doses of male sex hormones?

The Los Angeles County Medical Association's committee on sports medicine asked readers of *Muscle & Fitness* magazine, which has a circulation of about 800,000 and a readership of about three million, to write about personal experiences with steroids. Many of those who responded claimed to have experienced psychiatric effects.

One young woman wrote that she was troubled by horrible mood swings and was unable to sleep. She developed painful skin cysts on her back and chin, and her sex drive grew to embarrassing proportions. As aggressiveness increased, she "offered to punch out guys on the street." Although she has stopped taking steroids, she still has a baritone voice (she used to sing soprano) and excess facial hair. Worse, she has cystic breast disease and has been unable to conceive.

Although she has stopped taking steroids, she still has a baritone voice (she used to sing soprano) and excess facial hair.

Another woman had savage rages and no patience. Her outbursts became so uncontrolled that she was fired from her job and beat her boyfriend so badly he required medical attention.

These are frightening stories, even more so when you consider that the steroid-using population is varied and includes military personnel, police officers, and firefighters.

Charting Adverse Effects

Whether a steroid user is apt to have psychological effects is another matter. One convicted steroid dealer who served time in federal prison told us that he never knew any user to have the type of profound psychiatric effects now being described. However, there are reasons why that might be so. First, as a former elite athlete himself, he was among the first wave of steroid users who usually took smaller doses and fewer cycles than today's users. They were likely to inject drugs, whereas many users who face drug testing have switched to oral drugs or the esters of testosterone. Oral steroids appear to be more related to the occurrence of serious psychological or behavioral effects.

As a group, the first steroid users were older and began taking drugs at a later age than today's users do. Most were already competing at elite levels of sports, and their drug use was more goal-oriented. Some old-time users say that aggression or frank rage that might have accompanied drug taking was either channeled into doing the weight workout, or expressed away from the gym.

Why one person should be profoundly affected and another not at all is a mystery, but young users never know for certain their vulnerability. Dr. Pope says, "Acne will go away and testicles will resume their normal size, but if you're in jail for 20 years, that's a pretty serious adverse effect in itself."

Data from animal studies suggest that both androgens and estrogens bind to receptors in the nervous system that appear to selectively stimulate the nerve pathways associated with aggression. The question is: do increasing levels of testosterone result in more aggressive behavior, or does more aggressive behavior produce higher levels of testosterone? This question deserves further research. There have been attempts to link plasma testosterone levels with degrees of hostility or aggression. However, the results of those studies are equivocal.

Oral steroids appear to be more related to the occurrence of serious psychological or behavioral effects.

Drug dependency may be another problem for long-time steroid users, and the risk may be increased by taking higher doses or for longer periods of time. An article in the *Journal of the American Medical Association* in December 1989 suggested that there is a previously unrecognized form of drug addiction, a sex steroid hormone-dependence disorder. This disorder can be identified by certain criteria, according to the authors, Yale University psychiatrist Kenneth B. Kashkin, M.D., and Herbert D. Kleber, M.D., formerly at Yale and now the deputy to drug czar William Bennett:

- Use of the hormones continues over a longer period than desired or originally planned.

- Attempts to stop use are not successful.

- Substantial time is spent obtaining, using, or recovering from hormones.

- Hormone use continues despite knowledge of significant physical, psychological, or other personal problems caused by them.

- Characteristic drug withdrawal symptoms occur.

- Hormone use may be resumed to relieve the withdrawal symptoms.

"There appear to be similarities in the psychoactive properties of mood-altering substances of abuse and the steroid class of hormones," they wrote. They also said that the withdrawal syndromes are similar to those experienced by alcohol or cocaine users.

Not everyone agrees with the Kashkin/Kleber hypothesis. At Pennsylvania State, epidemiologist Charles Yesalis, Sc.D., says: "Although I find their hypothesis interesting, not one of the more than 200 elite and professional athletes I have interviewed has been unable to stop steroid use after they retired, which, of course, is inconsistent with the notion of biological addiction."

Physical Effects

The physical effects of steroid use also vary from user to user. What we can say with certainty and confidence about both general and specific adverse effects is that anabolic hormones are metabolized by and are capable of exerting effects on virtually every cell in the body. They do not act only on muscle tissue. One reason doctors believe that high doses of steroids are more risky is because they can stimulate the entire range of sex hormone receptors, so that the effects can include those that normally are seen with estrogens and progestins, and not just the androgens. The major organs and systems most likely to have altered functions include: the liver; the kidneys; the nervous, endocrine, and cardiovascular systems; the testes and other sex glands; and the spleen, lymph nodes and other cells and tissues of the immune system. The degree of derangement of body chemistry depends on whether the drug is taken by mouth or injection, by the dosage and length of use, and by interactions with other drugs being used simultaneously (Figure 3-1).

Anabolic hormones are metabolized by and capable of exerting effects on virtually every cell in the body. They do not act only on muscle tissue.

The liver is the body organ most likely to show effects of steroids since it is the primary means of clearing these drugs from the body. Sick people who take steroids for medical reasons sometimes get tumors or blood-filled cysts in the liver. These tumors do not have the characteristics of typical cancer and usually regress after drug use is discontinued. The cysts also resolve after drugs are stopped. There have been many anecdotal reports of liver damage in healthy athletes taking steroids. It does make sense that the liver would be damaged by steroid use, particularly now that so many athletes have switched to oral steroids because they wash out of the system faster than the oil-based injectables. Once Ben Johnson owned up to his past steroid use, he also admitted to having abnormal liver function tests.

Although some may think there have been many deaths from steroid-related liver tumors, that is not so. Karl Friedl, Ph.D., an Army captain at the Army Research Institute of Environmental Medicine, in Natick, Massachusetts, has done a

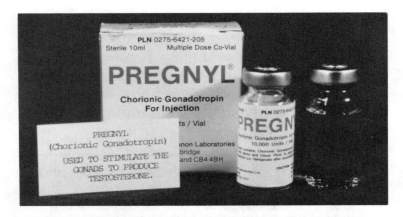

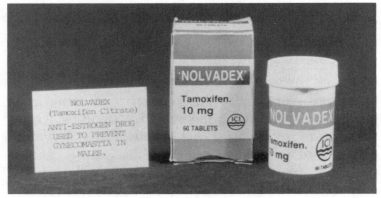

FIGURE 3-1. The drugs above are used with steroids to counteract unwanted effects. (Top) Pregnyl is one brand of human chorionic gonadotropin. It is a glycoprotein secreted by the placenta and obtained from the urine of pregnant women. It mimics luteinizing hormone in its stimulation of the interstitial cells of the testes, which increases production of testosterone. Athletes use it for many reasons, but primarily to increase the diminished androgen production and testicular size when coming off an episode of steroid use. It also increases natural testosterone levels prior to drug testing, and, during a steroid cycle, it is used in an attempt to maintain a better balance of androgens and estrogens. Reported side effects include allergic reactions, headaches, fatigue, mood changes, fluid retention, and gynecomastia. (Bottom) Nolvadex (one of several trade names for tamoxifen citrate) is an estrogen antagonist, used medically to stimulate ovulation and to treat some estrogen-sensitive cancers. Athletes use it to reduce the estrogenic effects caused by the body's conversion of some anabolic steroids to estrogens, in particular the development of gynecomastia.

computer search of the medical literature looking for liver tumors — and could find only three in athletes. There are 91 cases of androgen-associated tumors in the medical literature but some were not histologically confirmed and the rest were in sick people, not athletes.

In the three athletes, the first was a 27-year-old bodybuilder who used steroids for at least three years and who died of hemorrhage secondary to benign tumor rupture. The second patient was a 37-year-old athlete who used 100 mg a day of oxymetholone for five years. He is doing reasonably well after surgery. The third patient, a 26-year-old bodybuilder who was said to have used many androgens over a four-year period, had a tumor that was more consistent with classic liver cancer than with steroid-associated tumors. He developed metastatic disease and died within three months of diagnosis.

The liver is the body organ most likely to show effects of steroids since it is the primary means of clearing these drugs from the body.

Virtually all of the reported liver problems seem to occur with what are called the 17 alpha-alkylated steroids (steroids with a chemical group added to the number 17 carbon atom of the steroid skeleton). There have been no cysts or liver tumors reported in athletes who used the 17 beta-esterified injectable steroids. Whether former users will develop liver problems including tumors and cysts as they age is as yet unknown. Dr. Friedl noted that the absence of adverse effects in the medical literature does not mean they are not occurring, but he stresses the need for more scientific data and less anecdotal information. He has estimated that from 1 to 3 percent of individuals consuming greater than therapeutic doses of 17 alpha-alkylated steroids will develop liver tumors within two to eight years, although the latency period may be as long as 30 years, so that some users may never know about the tumors. Dr. Friedl suspects that some athletes may have benign tumors that remain undetected because they don't rupture and cause hemorrhage.

Another worrisome potential adverse effect to most steroid users is the possibility of dying from a heart attack or stroke.

Another worrisome potential adverse effect to most steroid users is the possibility of dying from a heart attack or stroke. What we can say for certain is that blood samples from anabolic steroids users frequently have high levels of the harmful low-density lipoprotein (LDL) cholesterol and lower levels of high-density lipoprotein (HDL). LDL cholesterol is the kind of fat that blocks the arteries around the heart, whereas HDL cholesterol is believed to help remove fat deposits from vessels. These changes are more likely to occur in oral steroid users.

Studies of animals have shown that anabolic steroids cause changes within the heart muscle itself, and some experts believe that these drugs may be a contributing factor in the development of cardiomyopathy in humans. Without long-term studies, we will not know if these temporary changes in blood fats or in the heart muscle resolve after steroid use is discontinued or whether they result in an increased incidence of heart attacks and other cardiovascular diseases.

Several steroid experts say they have information on heart attacks resulting in death that appeared to have at least a strong association with previous steroid use. These cases do not appear in the medical literature as steroid-related. Douglas McKeag, M.D., of Michigan State University, Lansing, has started a registry to collect data, and he has asked readers to notify him of deaths or serious illnesses that appear to be linked to steroid use.

Most people know about Steve Courson, a former lineman for the Pittsburgh Steelers and the Tampa Bay Bucaneers who is now awaiting a heart transplant and who believes his heart problems were caused by steroid use. Courson began taking the drugs as a 17-year-old player at the University of South Carolina and he continued using them when he went to the Steelers.

"They were so prevalent when I was in football that I looked at it as a tactical necessity..."

"They were so prevalent when I was in football that I looked at it as a tactical necessity," Courson has said.

As a professional player, Courson weighed 285 pounds and could bench press more than 580 pounds. He could run 40 yards in 4.6 seconds and had a 36-inch vertical leap. After leaving football, his weight increased to 310 pounds and he could bench press 605 pounds, a feat that made him one of the five strongest men in the world. He finished his football career in 1985. In November 1988, Courson felt ill and went to a Pittsburgh area hospital emergency room. The diagnosis was congestive heart failure and kidney and liver dysfunction. He notes that physicians aren't sure if his long-time use of steroids caused all the damage, but Courson believes that it is responsible.

Some may wonder why Courson's doctors don't just say flat out that steroids are the reason he needs a heart transplant. What we don't know is what Courson's genetic makeup and other habits may have contributed. A steroid user might die of a heart attack in his twenties, but if his father died of a heart attack at about the same age, it would be very difficult to prove the role, if any, of drugs as a cause of death.

Sports Illustrated ran an article in 1989 claiming that the death of an Ohio high school football player was the first to be officially linked to steroid use. There are several problems with this conclusion. First, there is no evidence that steroids caused his death. The autopsy results showed that the youth had a slightly enlarged heart and a viral disease, and the official cause of death was listed as viral endocarditis, not a myocardial infarction. Even the slightly enlarged heart cannot be definitely attributed to steroids since it is a common exercise-induced finding in athletes that usually has no clinical significance. Furthermore, even if steroids were a contributing cause in this young athlete's death, he was not the first to die from using steroids.

There are eight cases, including four deaths, in the medical literature of androgen-associated disease and undoubtedly there will be more as physicians make the association and report the cases. Dr. Friedl says that not all steroid-associated deaths will be recognized as such because athletes who have significant health problems may actually conceal their past drug use when they do seek medical help. In addition to the three liver tumors described earlier, the other five include:

- A 38-year-old bodybuilder who was a long-time user of high dose methandrostenolone died of Wilm's tumor, a rare cancer of the kidney, in 1977.

- A 40-year-old bodybuilder died of prostate cancer after using 15 or more cycles of many androgens over a 20-year period.

- A 34-year-old bodybuilder who used numerous cycles of anabolic steroids over a four-year period has made a partial recovery after suffering a stroke.

- A 32-year-old bodybuilder who used many androgens since the age of 16 has made a partial recovery from blockage of a blood vessel in the brain but he now has heart damage.

- A 22-year-old power lifter who weighed 330 pounds used oral and injected androgens for a six-week period before suffering a heart attack. He has since recovered.

Increases in blood pressure readings occur in some users. Among the possible reasons are increased fluid retention, altered metabolism, or enhanced production or secretion of corticosteroids from the adrenal glands. The increases in blood pressure generally tend to be small, inconsistent, and unpredictable, but may be dramatic at times.

At least one investigator believes that using androgens may pose a risk of blood clots. We know that there are changes in the clotting factor with the 17 alpha-alkylated steroids, and that there are several medical reports of strokes in patients and athletes using steroids. It may be that the steroids that are aromatized (converted into estrogen-like products) might cause a slight increase in the risk of stroke, but that has not been demonstrated conclusively.

Steroid effects on the reproductive system can be complicated. When sex hormones from outside the body are taken, the brain signals the body to lessen its production of sex hormones in an effort to keep everything in balance.

Steroid effects on the reproductive system can be complicated.

Without the natural production, sperm production diminishes in men and usually ceases altogether after a time. The testicles shrink in size even though sexual interest maybe enhanced for some period of time. Richard Strauss, M.D., a steroid expert at Ohio State, has said that the effect of steroids on sex drive is highly variable. A common pattern, according to Dr. Strauss, is for the sex drive to increase when steroids are begun, then decrease to normal or below normal after several weeks. Some users never notice any changes, but some men who used steroids for prolonged periods believe their sex drive never returned to normal after they stopped using the drugs.

The large amounts of male sex hormones in the body (from outside sources) may be broken down

into other substances that are similar to e
a female sex hormone, so that men develop
and their voices get higher. Women, on tl
hand, will have lower voices (a permanen
tion), shrinking of breast tissue, enlarged genitals,
and unwanted facial and body hair growth. We do
not know whether all former steroid users — both
male and female — who later wish to have children
will be able to or whether sterility may result in at
least a small percentage of users. Medical literature contains no reports of permanent sterility in
male steroid users who had normal sperm counts
when they began using drugs.

There have been anecdotal reports from East
Germany that at least one of the women swimmers
who used steroids could not conceive and that
another has a physically handicapped child. There
is some question about whether taking sex hormones for long periods might interfere with the
rhythms of natural hormones. As people age, the
rhythm of hormone production changes anyway.
The question is whether disrupting that normal
rhythmic process by taking steroids over a long
period might prevent a return to normal, and perhaps even accelerate the aging process.

Steroids suppress the body's immune system,
so that some experts have speculated that this
might affect resistance to disease and recovery
from bacterial and viral infections, and perhaps
even the development of various cancers.

When young boys take anabolic steroids, one
of the main dangers of which we are aware is that
the growth plates on the ends of their bones may
close prematurely so that their adult height is
shorter than it would have been. However, adoles-

cent boys are already undergoing a natural surge of testosterone. Whether adding a flood of synthetic sex hormones to this natural production may cause special vulnerability is a question for future research. We believe this user group may be more vulnerable to permanent damage from anabolic steroid use. — *adolescents*

When young boys take anabolic steroids, one of the main dangers of which we are aware is that growth plates on the ends of their bones may close permanently so that their adult height is shorter than it would have been.

Still another area that needs investigation is drug interactions, including whether steroids may be a gateway for other drug use. Individuals who use heavy cycles of steroids often increase their consumption of sedatives or hypnotics. Some users say they increase their alcohol or marijuana consumption while they are on a steroid cycle to reduce the arousal caused by the intense training and steroids. One former world record holder in power lifting used to drink a six-pack of beer at the end of each day to "come down." Other drugs may carry their own special health risks. Obviously, there are unknown interactive effects that come from combining anabolic steroids with other drugs, and these may potentiate changes in behavior patterns.

Some have wondered if alcohol could be a trigger for violent behavior in steroid users. There is a case from Canada in which a 32-year-old amateur bodybuilder and steroid user with no previous history of criminal behavior or psychiatric problems was convicted of the second-degree murder of his common law wife, after heavy drinking recollection, he was taking six tablets (mg) of Dianabol a day orally and half Deca-Durabolin (either 50 or 100 mg) by once a week. His friends at the gym where he trained told him there were no adverse effects. Some four weeks before the crime, he became nervous, irritable, and had difficulty sleeping. He drank alcohol to cope with these symptoms. On the night of the crime, both he and his wife were drinking heavily. When she confessed to being unfaithful, he beat her so severely that she died of head injuries. Six months after the crime, the man was again mentally normal.

Alcohol is known to be associated with reduced inhibitions and violent and aggressive behavior. In this particular case, it is important to note what seem to be interactive effects between the steroids and alcohol so that there were frank personality changes and a greater degree of expressed violence.

Two other adverse effects that seem almost minor in comparison to some of the potentially serious consequences are acne and hair loss. Acne may cover the upper arms, shoulders, and backs of heavy users, as well as the face. Hair loss is often rapid and usually is most prominent at the top rear of the head and in a receding hairline just above the temples.

An increased susceptibility to connective tissue injuries is another potential problem for steroid users. Animal studies, medical case reports of tendon and ligament damage in strength athletes, and anecdotal reports from athletes all give credence to this possibility.

We have not always separated men and women in talking about health effects, but we should note that all women who take anabolic steroids will suffer some irreversible masculinizing effects. A woman's physical appearance may be completely altered. Television viewers of the Olympic Games of the 1970s became accustomed to seeing masculine-looking women from the Eastern Bloc countries. There was suspicion that they were men in women's clothes, but they were undoubtedly women taking steroids. Besides the irreversible masculinization, women have the same health risks from steroid use as men.

Two other adverse effects that seem almost minor in comparison to some of the potentially serious consequences are acne and hair loss.

Research is urgently needed to identify and quantify the risks associated with the use of anabolic steroids, including those of undesirable or antisocial behavior, and the long-term health risks. We need to know if these risks are increased by age, dosages of drugs, and length of administration. It may be another decade before any answers are forthcoming. If the present rate of steroid use continues, the number of individuals at risk for adverse effects will much greater than it is today.

4

RECOGNIZING ANABOLIC STEROID USE

A large urban high school recently added a young man to its internal security force. A teacher who had known the new employee during his student days at the high school took one look at the physical transformation that had taken place since he had last seen him and called it to the attention of an administrator. Pointing out the almost unbelievable muscular development and definition, he stated his conviction that the young man was using anabolic steroids, and asked how he could be considered a good role model for students.

"Well, we asked him if he took steroids," was the reply, "and he said no."

Why are we not surprised? Steroid taking is a very secretive behavior. Charles Yesalis, Sc.D., of Pennsylvania State University, said at a Maryland seminar on steroids that athletes would sooner confess to using cocaine than they would anabolic steroids. He added that secrecy must be a methodological consideration for researchers. People who use steroids talk about it openly only with other users. There is a steroid-user subculture.

Steroid taking is a very secretive behavior...athletes would sooner confess to using cocaine than they would anabolic steroids.

If we can't just ask, then there must be other signs and symptoms that raise the index of suspicion. The most obvious clues to anabolic steroid use are rapid increases in strength and/or size beyond what could be expected from ordinary training. When a teenager appears to put on 10 to 20 pounds of solid muscle in a relatively brief period of time — six weeks to two months — parents, coaches, or trainers should be alert to the possibility that steroids are being used, particularly if the weight gain is accompanied by mood changes. Weight gain does not occur in all steroid users, so other signs and symptoms must also be examined.

Many adolescent boys and girls begin training with weights somewhere between the ages of 12 and 15 years, and nearly all high school sports programs include some form of weight work. Good weight training can enhance the development of size (mainly in males) and produce gains in muscular strength and endurance in both males and females. Performance in almost any sport may be enhanced by regular weight workouts, provided the program was designed by someone familiar with the physical demands of the sport and the athlete's potential for improvement and commitment to the program.

In an unknown number of adolescents and young adults, weight training appears to precipitate a change of focus so that as changes occur in the body because of the training, the changed body becomes the goal in itself instead of just part of the preparation to participate in sports. Some youths begin weight training with the goal of attaining a powerful physique and may never be involved in individual or team sports. For whatever reason training is undertaken, whenever an adolescent or young adult becomes totally immersed in changing his body, a caution flag should be raised.

The perception of reality in steroid users — especially with regard to body image — may be equally as diminished as it is in people with anorexia.

Several experts have suggested, and we agree, that "bulking up" may be the other side of anorexia nervosa and that many of the same basic drives exist in both. The perception of reality in steroid users - especially with regard to body image - may be equally diminished as it is in people with anorexia. We are certainly not suggesting that everyone who wants to go into weight lifting or bodybuilding has a problem. We agree with Don Leggett, a drug expert at the Food and Drug Administration.

"Bulging muscles are in," he said. "Guys want to look good at the beach. High-school kids think steroids may enhance their ability to get an athletic scholarship, play pro sports or win the girl of their heart. Steroid use in this country has spread down to general people."

Signs and Symptoms

Steroid use may have spread to general people but most don't know what signs to look for. John Lombardo, M.D., a sports medicine expert at the Cleveland Clinic Foundation in Ohio, put together a list of warning signs of drug use in the young steroid abuser. These include:

- Being involved in activities where steroid use is known to flourish

- The amount of weight and size that is gained over a short period of time

- Changes in behavior

- Physical signs, including hair loss, acne, or breast development in males

- Changes in laboratory data taken as part of a physical examination.

Historically, sports that rely on weight training as the main form of conditioning have been the activities most likely to lead to anabolic steroid use. Football, weight lifting (Olympic or power), the track and field sports, and bodybuilding are activities where adolescents and young men and women are apt to come into contact with users of anabolic steroids. However, steroids have also been detected in many seemingly unlikely sports, including swimming and distance running where their use allows athletes to perform more frequent and higher-intensity workouts rather than to increase weight or strength.

There may be many paths of initiation to anabolic steroids, but many younger athletes obviously come in contact with seasoned users through their sports activities. In power lifting, for instance, a younger person may work out with an experienced lifter. Dr. Lombardo says the same situation exists in bodybuilding, a sport that requires size, muscle definition, and the ability to perform frequent high-intensity workouts. He notes that weight lifters are another group that is very sensitive to physical appearance.

In sports like football, the primary motivating factor for steroid use is more likely to be the obvious financial and social rewards that come with success, rather than simply a desire to look different. Many young football players train at local gyms during the summer where they talk with power lifters and bodybuilders who may introduce the subject of steroid use. Football players know that size is intimidating and that physical size usually is equated with power. Size is self-reinforcing. Nobody who is big (muscular) ever wants to be smaller. College football players key on gains in size and strength to estimate when an opponent has added anabolic steroids to his program. They also know that in professional football, most of the players are on a nearly equal footing in terms of physical talent and technique. Increasing size is one way they can increase their perceived strength and power and attract the attention of a National Football League team. In their zeal to play professional football, young players often rationalize their drug use, says Dr. Lombardo.

The field events — particularly those requiring great strength, the discus, shot-put, and hammer throw — have had more than their share of anabolic steroid abuse. Younger athletes who compete in these events will come into contact with older athletes, some of whom will undoubtedly have used steroids.

There may be many paths of initiation to anabolic steroids, but many younger athletes obviously come in contact with seasoned users through their sports activities.

Quick gains in size and strength may be the number one indicator of steroid use, but another important symptom that is likely to be noticed by an athlete's family is a change in appetite. The legendary eating feats of teenagers could fill a separate book, either on nutrition or humor, and the fact that an adolescent boy eats as a snack the roast that was prepared for dinner does not, in itself, mean he is a steroid user. However, if that adolescent has been eating six to eight ounces of meat at a meal but now consumes 12 to 16 ounces of meat at a sitting, day after day, something may be amiss. An anabolic steroid user may continue to fill his plate long after other family members have finished, or he may eat more or less constantly rather than at specified meals. At the same time, the person may be very particular about his diet, even count calories or insist on certain types and amounts of food. When an adolescent increases food intake substantially but does not become overweight, parents must assess the situation.

Increased appetite may be harder to gauge when the user does not live at home. A college training table is expected to hold generous amounts of food, and if even that amount is supplemented by snacks elsewhere, who is going to know?

Acne is a noticeable and common sign of steroid use, particularly if it appears on the upper back, shoulders, and arms as well as the face. Some steroid users develop a puffy appearance, especially around their faces, or they look as if their tissues are retaining fluid. Still another clue is premature male pattern baldness, including a rapidly receding hairline, loss of hair from the top rear of the head, or hair loss in patches. Because this hair loss may be dramatic, parents might simply check the drain in the shower or tub.

When an adolescent increases food intake substantially but does not become overweight, parents must assess the situation.

A change in sleep patterns, especially if a young person seems to have plenty of energy but needs less sleep than before could signal steroid use, particularly if it occurs in combination with other signs. However, it must also be kept in mind that harder training can increase sleep needs and possibly mask steroid effects. Also, overexertion or overtraining can affect sleep habits dramatically.

An increase in moodiness — or sudden shifts in mood — are another important indicator. Perfectly normal teenagers undergo profound and sometimes rapid changes of mood because of the increased production of their own natural hormones, and it may be difficult to tell when those shifts are being augmented by the addition of synthetic hormones. When mood shifts are characterized by irritability, hostility, or aggressiveness, the index of suspicion may be raised if other symptoms of drug use are present.

Mood changes are easier to identify in young adults whose natural hormonal upheavals have quieted down. Anabolic steroid use may produce elevated moods, euphoria, and an increased sense of well-being, self-confidence, and self- esteem, particularly if the individual is pleased with his gains in size, strength, appearance, and performance.

When mood shifts are characterized by irritability, hostility, or aggressiveness, the index of suspicion may be raised if other symptoms of drug use are present.

Adult steroid users may experience an increase, at least temporarily, in sexual interest. However, that interest may be displayed more aggressively. Many of the mood states of steroid users contain a component of aggression. It may be directed toward people or objects, and it may take either verbal or physical form. A study of hockey players (who were not steroid users) showed that their response to perceived threat was strongly associated with naturally elevated testosterone levels. Aggressiveness on the playing field is generally a trait prized by coaches, but if the aggressive behavior extends to friends, at home, or in school, take a second look.

Everyone experiences hormonal changes at times, and these shifts sometimes cause dramatic changes in mood. The most common natural sex hormone-related mood changes occur in women during the premenstrual period. Many women report high levels of anxiety and irritability during the stage of the monthly cycle when estrogen, progesterone, and androgen levels are fluctuating. Men experience the same type of symptoms when, for varying reasons such as aging, illness, and stress, their levels of testosterone fluctuate. These mood shifts have been felt to some degree by almost every adult man and woman. Anabolic steroid users may experience very exaggerated changes of mood and may even have a hard time maintaining emotional control. The net result is that any shifts in mood — up, down, or rapidly fluctuating — that are not normal for a particular person are cause for concern.

Lowering of the voice or growth of body hair can be signs of anabolic steroid use that would be unremarkable in adolescent boys, but conspicuous in young women. Boys may have enlargement of breast tissue seen usually as a protruding appearance around the nipples. This means that metabolic changes have occurred, increasing estrogen levels and stimulating the growth of breast tissue. Breast enlargement sometimes occurs naturally in boys going through puberty, although it almost always resolves within a short time.

Lowering of the voice or growth of body hair can be signs of anabolic steroid use that would be unremarkable in adolescent boys, but conspicuous in young women.

On the other hand, a young woman who has started taking steroids will lose her breast tissue and her chest will look more manly. She probably will experience some form of menstrual disturbance such as painful or absent periods. Her skin may become coarse and rough and hairy. Dr. Lombardo says that the time span during which symptoms appear varies with the drug used, its dosage, and the length of time it is taken, but if the drug contains testosterone, masculinization will occur very quickly.

One noticeable physical sign of testosterone use in both sexes is reddening of the face, neck, and upper chest region so they appear constantly flushed. This reddening is more obvious in the winter, but the flushed area can still be observed in the summer as redder or darker skin. Steroid users may try to pass it off as simply too much sun exposure, but the pattern is suggestive of drug use.

Jaundice, or yellowing of the skin or the whites of the eyes, is another sign that will be obvious in both men and women. It signals serious disturbance of liver function when it occurs.

A clue to drug use that might be observed more quickly at home is the possession of unusual pills, vials, syringes, or paraphernalia associated with injections, such as alcohol pads or parts of syringes. Parents do have a legal right to search their child's possessions, but most would see that step only as a last resort because of the nearly inevitable breach of good relations between parent and child such a search would bring about.

Speaking Up

Once anabolic steroid use is suspected, the next question is: what should be done about it? If the signs and symptoms of drug use appear to be minimal and the user does not seem to have any adverse effects, there may be a temptation to do nothing, particularly if the user is a successful athlete. For several important reasons, this is not the correct course of action.

First, anabolic steroid use is unethical. In fact, many steroid experts view steroid use as primarily an ethical problem rather than a health issue. When this form of cheating is accepted or tolerated by family, friends, teammates, coaches, or others, it sends a message to the user that cheating is okay. It erodes the values of those who do it and those who allow it. Almost as important for the individual is the fact that when there is an overwhelming preoccupation with body image, the emotional, spiritual, and intellectual sides of personality may be neglected, leaving a one-dimensional person who is incapable of the normal give and take of life. Further, this person may begin relying on drugs in place of coping skills and self-esteem once he gets too far behind in the other areas.

What parent really wants his child to serve as a guinea pig in an uncontrolled experiment with potentially dangerous drugs?

Second, anabolic steroid use may cause health problems.What parent really wants his child to serve as a guinea pig in an uncontrolled experiment with potentially dangerous drugs? Would you permit a healthy youngster to participate in a clinical trial of a new medicine that might have both short- and long-term harmful effects on his health? Whatever the underground steroid literature may say, the health risks have not been calculated. As David R. Lamb, Ph.D., a professor at Ohio State University, has said: "It is hard to believe that such powerful drugs will not have damaging side effects with prolonged use...."

Moreover, the youngest users may be more vulnerable to damage because their bodies are still developing and some systems may not yet be mature. Their bodies are just beginning to produce adult sex hormones, and taking them in from outside may cause far-reaching and, as yet unknown, hazards. Besides the physical immaturity, these youngsters are also in a delicate transitional state emotionally and psychologically, a state that could be disrupted by drugs.

Yet another reason to take action where steroid use is suspected is that many users obtain their drugs on the black market.

Another reason to confront steroid use is the fact that new users may be making a long-term commitment to drugs. Paul Goldstein, Ph.D., spoke about the natural progression of steroid use at a National Institute of Drug Abuse (NIDA) consensus conference on steroids. The first stage is one of exploration, followed by a continuation stage where use of steroids is regular. The third stage is stopping use, a step many cannot take until their health is threatened. Because anabolic steroids improve, at least initially, the sense of well being of those that take them, drug-taking behavior is reinforced. Users may be pleased with the way their steroid-enhanced bodies look, and they fail to realize that they will lose both size and strength when that use is discontinued. How much size and strength is lost is another unanswered question but it appears to be enough to keep many steroid users (perhaps as many as 75 percent) on the drugs for years. Youngsters who take anabolic steroids are, in effect, walking down a blind alley filled with moral and physical potholes.

Yet another reason to take action where steroid use is suspected is that many users obtain their drugs on the black market. The purity of these preparations is suspect. Unless drugs are obtained from companies that are required to maintain sterility and purity, there is no way to be assured of what the buyer is actually purchasing. The uncontrolled drugs may contain inert substances. They may have been made in unclean surroundings, and users may be putting unknown or harmful counterfeit substances in their bodies. Injections carry the risk of infection or hepatitis, and there have been at least two reported cases of transmission of AIDS through shared needles.

What To Do

If a parent suspects that his child may be using anabolic steroids and the relationship is such that he can ask, that is the appropriate course of action. The conversation with the child should be non-judgmental in tone and convey the clear message that the parent is concerned for the health and emotional well-being of the user. The next step is to determine the length of use, the dosage, where the supply is being obtained, and the stated reason for use. If that use is anything more than a casual, experimental event, a parent would be wise to seek professional advice.

If a parent thinks his child is using anabolic steroids and cannot be sure his child would tell the truth about it, an initial course of action might be to arrange an appointment with a physician for a complete physical. The doctor will be able to order basic tests to assess liver function and blood fat levels, examine the patients for acne and edema, and check males for testicle size and consistency.

If a male user is also taking human chorionic gonadotropin along with the steroids, his testicles may be of normal size. Another drug some users take to maintain normal testicle size is clomiphene citrate. This drug, which is used to induce ovulation in women, is taken at the end of a steroid cycle. It is an estrogen receptor blocker, and it "fools" the pituitary gland into secreting gonadotropins.

Other conditions a doctor may see in a male steroid user, particularly a long-time user, include prostatic hypertrophy, a condition in which the prostate enlarges and presses on the surrounding vessels so that there is difficulty in voiding. The prostate gland may resume its normal size when drugs are stopped.

Youngsters who take anabolic steroids are, in effect, walking down a blind alley filled with moral and physical potholes.

Blood pressure may have risen enough that frank hypertension is present. However, blood pressure increases also have been reported by strength-training athletes who don't use steroids, and this phenomenon may accompany overtraining in any activity.

Concerned parents should understand their physician's views and recommendations for treatment before making an appointment for their child.

Not all doctors will recognize the signs of anabolic steroid use. Some doctors will feel uncomfortable discussing that issue with a patient. They may be too judgmental or authoritarian in their approach. Moreover steroid users seldom trust physicians and usually have discounted them as sources of reliable information about steroids. While many doctors have studied the steroid literature, there still are physicians who believe that anabolic steroids are simply an expensive placebo. Still other physicians view steroid use as an individual choice (although we know that far fewer prescriptions are being written for them now, reflecting a change of attitude about health risks).

Concerned parents should understand their physician's views and recommendations for treatment before making an appointment for their child.

Sometimes parents remain unaware of steroid abuse when an athletic trainer, coach, or team member may suspect it. If the relationship is close, one of these individuals may be in an excellent position to express concern in such a way that the athlete is moved to discontinue use, or to get help if he is unable to stop on his own.

What makes steroid users stop is something we know little about. Several long-term users say that if a person stays on steroids a year, he is on them for life. However, there are many instances where an athlete stopped steroids when he retired from competition, with apparently little physical or psychological difficulty.

Paul Goldstein, Ph.D., a speaker at the 1989 National Institute of Drug Abuse consensus conference on steroids, said there seem to be two prominent reasons for stopping. Young persons, Goldstein said, mature to a point where career, marriage, and conventional lifestyles are more highly valued than the macho image of great strength and size. Older steroid users tend to quit only when their health is seriously threatened. Goldstein believes there is a third group of users who are goal-directed in their drug use so that, once they achieve their goal or move on, they discontinue drugs. Perhaps many elite athletes fit this third category.

When an athlete is goal-directed, a coach or trainer may influence him by showing him other legitimate ways to achieve his end. A coach also is in a position to apply sanctions for continued use. These sanctions need not be severe, just strong enough to convey the message that steroid use is unacceptable. Some experts suggest a warning for a first steroid offense, followed by a very strong penalty if there is a second.

Substance Abuse Problem?

When an athlete has been confronted about his abuse of steroids and when sanctions have not been successful in deterring use, it would be wise to seek the assistance of a professional in the field of substance abuse treatment. This could be a social worker, psychologist, or psychiatrist, but it should be someone who has dealt with steroid users. Some psychotherapists believe that steroid abuse should be treated in the same way as any other substance abuse problem. They say that it has the same common features as any other addiction. Treatment may be difficult and not always successful, and relapses can be expected. A psychologist at a private psychiatric hospital near Chicago said he has treated two steroid users but was able to help only one of them. The second patient was completely unwilling to remain in treatment and has gone back to using steroids.

Not all steroid users become dependent on the drugs, of course, and one reason to consider a psychological evaluation is to discover whether dependence has developed or is likely to. Rehabilitation is indicated for steroid users who have serious health problems related to their drug use, or for users who have developed psychological dependence. This does not mean that others should not stop taking steroids, but some people who have used them simply stop voluntarily and without any apparent ill effects.

Some users who "stack" drugs — meaning they take several different kinds of steroids and other drugs in a patterned use — may experience a broader range of symptoms when disorders do occur. The theory behind stacking is that combination of drugs give a better result than the same dose of just one drug. Also, users believe that the effects on body organs are not as stressful when more than one type of drug is used. Most users combine oral and injected drugs.

Kirk J. Brower, M.D., a psychiatrist at the University of Michigan, presented a paper on rehabilitation at a consensus meeting on steroids held in Los Angeles in July 1989. He has divided steroids users into three groups: the athlete, the person for whom looking fit is more important than being fit, and a third group he calls the "fighting elite," which includes soldiers, bouncers, law enforcement officers, and street gang members. This third group is interested in physical power. The common theme underlying all three groups, according to Dr. Brower, is an over-reliance on physical attributes to obtain a sense of self-worth. (Athletes would undoubtedly defend themselves by saying that academic types have an over-reliance on intellectual attributes for their sense of self-worth.)

...ultimately, rehabilitation may depend on the user's ability to identify sources of self-esteem other than physical appearance.

Most of the theories of how steroid dependence develops are speculative. We know there are steroid receptors in the brain but we don't know exactly where they are. It may be that when brain receptors are continually saturated, they become supersensitive and crave the drug. Another theory is that when steroids are stopped, testosterone levels fall and the withdrawal symptoms correspond to a testosterone deficiency. The effects of steroids on the electrical activity of the brain are comparable to those of stimulants and anti-depressants. Thus, it shouldn't be surprising that eliminating the drugs may result in a depressed state of mind, particularly when the user can see his body and physical capacities also wither.

Dr. Brower says that no matter the mechanism of dependence, many symptoms will be identical to other drug dependencies. Suicidal depressions can occur during withdrawal, and Dr. Brower thinks, for this reason alone, close professional monitoring is required when users with dependence problems discontinue steroids.

Former users can expect to experience strong desires to resume steroid use. Dr. Goldstein says that many of the conversational interchanges among steroids users are drug oriented. For example: Two men meeting at a gym in New York City exchanged greetings and one who had just returned from skiing remarked, "I can't wait to get back on the stuff."

When users want to maintain weight training but discontinue steroid use, it may be especially difficult for them because of the strong psychological and social pressure to resume. Dr. Brower said that, ultimately, rehabilitation may depend on the user's ability to identify sources of self-esteem other than physical appearance. That may be difficult because muscular development and strength are equated with sexual attractiveness.

Former users can expect to experience strong desires to resume steroid use.

Once abstinence from steroids is achieved, urine testing can be a tool to detect relapses and monitor abstinence. However, surprisingly, urine testing for steroids is not readily available to clinicians. The expense of gathering and maintaining metabolic pattern libraries and of training laboratory personnel are considerations that keep most commercial laboratories out of steroid drug testing. Although it is possible to arrange for steroid tests with one of the sports drug-testing laboratories, they are wary about accepting samples from unknown sources. They know it could be a case of an athlete wanting a "preview" before he underwent real drug testing.

Is It Your Problem?

A coach or trainer who suspects an athlete is using anabolic steroids is in a somewhat different position than a family member, particularly if the user is a high school or junior high school student. Colleges and elite sports programs generally have written provisions for dealing with actual or suspected steroid use and abuse. The National Collegiate Athletic Association (NCAA) has taken a leading role in promoting steroid education and drug testing at the collegiate level.

However, some high school coaches may prefer to keep their suspicions about an athlete to themselves simply because they do not know what steps to take. One urban physical education chairman said: "I would definitely confront the user and I would talk with his coach and with his parents. So far as a penalty goes, I don't know exactly what to say. We have not defined what the penalty for use should be."

That is probably not an uncommon position. High school coaches are just coming to the point of dealing with spreading use. They are beginning to recognize that just as recreational drug use spreads through a team, so does anabolic steroid use. However, most steroid abuse policies at the high school and junior high level have not been defined. Where they exist, high school policies and programs for handling steroid abuse vary from none to very good.

As might be expected, the programs are better in states where there are known to be large numbers of steroid users. Justin Cunningham, the health and physical education coordinator of the San Diego County Office of Education, is part of a group working to develop a steroid curriculum for the State of California, and he sees differences between steroid and recreational drug users.

"We don't see as much steroid activity in the lower socioeconomic groups out here," he reported. "We're finding kids in affluent neighborhoods are taking steroids."

Cunningham said that a survey of steroid use in California high schools showed that close to 40 percent of users listed appearance as their reason for taking steroids, and another 8 to 9 percent listed social reasons.

We should not be surprised at this, given that our society is full of explicit and hidden messages that physical attractiveness is necessary to success. Many commercial messages give the impression that taking certain drugs and eating certain foods are the way to be happy and healthy. When over-the-counter drugs are advertised on television and in magazines, the overriding message is that you have to supplement nature. Many anabolic steroid users see their use in just that light. The legal drugs of our society — alcohol, tobacco, and caffeine — have been successfully associated with having "fun" or being successful, and in that context, many regard steroids as just another success-oriented product.

5

DRUG TESTING

One day each week of the school year, between 15 and 30 student athletes at
Homewood-Flossmoor High School find their con-
fidential athlete numbers posted on a board. It is
Drug Testing Day at this large high school in an
affluent suburb south of Chicago. A reminder is
broadcast over the public address system at the
start of classes. The numbers of students to be
tested came from a random drawing conducted the
previous evening by Athletic Director Kenneth
Shultz and the head coach of at least one of the 24
sports offered at the school. After the first drawing,
two of those numbers are randomly selected for
steroid testing (at a different laboratory).

At a designated time, students report to a
locker room near the school stadium where they
are met by a medical team from an area hospital.
Each student must show the photograph on his or
her school ID card for verification of identity. Next
they fill out brief forms that include a description
of any over-the-counter and prescription medications they are taking. Then they remove their

clothes and don hospital gowns. A same-sex nurse accompanies each student to a toilet stall and stands on the other side of the partition while the student voids. (The toilet bowl contains a blueing agent to prevent dilution of the sample.) The sample is sealed and marked by the athlete and the collection person. The two students selected for steroid testing seal and mark the additional vials. Then each student athlete continues the otherwise typical routine of high school.

The process of testing is conducted under strict regulation and will be described later in this chapter. Parents of students with positive tests have the right to take a portion of the urine specimen to a laboratory of their choice for retesting. Test results are kept private. The school drug counselor has the responsibility of dealing with students who have positive drug tests, and sanctions may vary.

The program at Homewood-Flossmoor is the outgrowth of concern about how to identify and help students who might be abusing drugs. It appears to be well accepted by both parents and students, well thought out in its conception by the school administration, and well executed in a fair and honest way. The American Civil Liberties Union, which has actively intervened in some university drug testing venues by mounting legal challenges, has indicated it will not object so long as the testing is limited to athletes. (The Homewood-Flossmoor program is also discussed in the chapter on legal issues).

Shultz has been contacted by more than 250 high schools across the nation, and many of callers are interested in starting their own programs. However, before high school drug testing goes further, there are important points that should be discussed at length.

- Should high school students be subjected to drug testing at all?

- Is high school testing practical?

- Should athletes be singled out for drug testing?

- How reliable is the drug testing?

- Who will pay the admittedly high cost?

- What is the purpose of testing: to guarantee fair competition or to ensure the health and safety of the students?

The Era of Drug Testing

Drug testing in sports has been a fact of life for more than 20 years, since the 1968 Olympic Winter Games in Grenoble. Even so, there is still strong ambivalence about drug testing in the United States. This ambivalence relates to concerns about unconstitutional invasion of the privacy of the individual tested, the accuracy of the tests (both for false positives and false negatives), the rumors that some athletic organizations suppress positive tests, and justifying the costs of testing.

There is some sentiment that professional athletes who make a living from competing in sports should be allowed to make up their own minds about using performance-enhancing drugs. Others believe professional athletes are most vulnerable to coercion to use drugs. Until the past year, testing high school or younger students has not even been considered.

A separate point that must be examined is whether anabolic steroid use by adolescents and young adults who are not athletes and thus not subject to athlete drug testing will increase or remain at the same level in the absence of testing. This question is likely to remain unanswered for the foreseeable future. It is unlikely that there will be any testing of non-athlete high school students for anabolic steroid abuse unless (or until) a cheap, reliable drug test is developed.

Announced, one-time tests are useless because they give the public appearance of concern, while privately making it very easy for drug users to avoid detection.

We can speculate that young people who take steroids not for performance enhancement but for improved body image might be more likely to develop dependency problems than young athletes who are performance-directed in their drug use. If that should prove to be the case, the present drug testing would not identify the people most at risk.

We know enough about drug testing at this point to say that random, unannounced drug testing works to reduce (but not eliminate) drug use, particularly if it can be conducted on a year-round basis. Announced, one-time tests are useless because they give the public appearance of concern, while privately making it very easy for drug users to avoid detection.

Drug testing technology has become much more sophisticated, and the laboratories that are approved by the International Olympic Committee (IOC) are without peer. There are two IOC-approved laboratories in the United States: one at UCLA in Los Angeles, and the other at Indiana University in Indianapolis. A third highly regarded sports drug testing laboratory is located at Vanderbilt University in Nashville, Tennessee. Below that level, there are some good commercial laboratories and some that are not so good. However, all U.S. laboratories must now be approved by at least one of several professional organizations, or by an arm of the federal government.

It costs a lot of money to equip a first-class drug identification laboratory and to train its personnel. The Los Angeles Olympic Organizing Committee gave UCLA a grant of $1.8 million to set up the Paul Ziffren Olympic Analytical Facility to do the testing for the 1984 Olympic Games. It took about $2 million to set up the laboratory in Indianapolis and train the personnel to do the drug testing for the 1987 Pan American Games.

Drug Testing Policy

The most influential figure in U.S. sports drug testing is undoubtedly Don H. Catlin, M.D., director of the UCLA laboratory and a member of the Medical Commission of the International Olympic Committee (IOC). For a number of years he was chairman of the Substance Abuse Committee of the U.S. Olympic Committee, a post that has been taken over for this quadrennium by hurdler Edwin Moses.

In a recent interview with Dr. Catlin, he noted that number of high school students at risk is huge and that the expense of testing remains so high that only the most affluent school districts can even consider doing it. At present, steroid tests cost between $100 and $200. Although that figure can be expected to come down some as the number of tests increases, cost will continue to be a factor for some time.

"The demand for the type work we do is lower and the cost is high," Dr. Catlin said several years ago. "The only way to run efficiently is to have a lot of samples."

The expense of testing remains so high that only the most affluent school districts can even consider doing it.

However, broad-scale high school testing would involve too many samples at present. For instance, someone called Dr. Catlin recently for a cost estimate on testing 550,000 high school student athletes in California. Dr. Catlin explained that even in 1988 (an Olympic year) only 48,000 tests for anabolic steroids were done worldwide. Expense then becomes irrelevant.

Given these figures, it becomes immediately apparent that high school drug testing is neither practical nor economical for most school districts. About one million students play high school football, and steroid expert Dr. Yesalis of Pennsylvania State University has estimated the cost of testing each of them once a year at more than $100 million.

One reason the Homewood-Flossmoor High School program has been well received is because no tax dollars are used to support it. Athletic Director Shultz said the hospital picks up a portion of the estimated $50,000 yearly tab. An anonymous donor subsidized nearly half the first year's cost.

The school takes $1 out of every athletic ticket and puts that money in a special drug testing fund. If a shortfall occurs, the PTA and Athletic Booster Club plan to raise funds to cover it.

The question of who will pay for high school testing is important. Will it be a privilege of middle class suburban children? What happens if one community can afford to foot the bill and another can't? If we cannot guarantee that all high school, or college, or international athletes are drug free, can we guarantee that competition will be fair? Many coaches claim to have tolerated or encouraged steroid use so their athletes would compete on a "level playing field."

If we cannot guarantee that all high school, or college, or international athletes are drug free, can we guarantee that the competition will be fair?

"Massive education should be our first line of defense," says Dr. Catlin. "I also believe that we should target scarce resources for where we have reason to be concerned."

He is frequently called by school administrators or team physicians around the country, with most of the calls prompted by an actual case involving steroids. Somewhat surprisingly, Dr. Catlin says he still views testing as "an experimental tool." Rather than plunging into broad scale high school testing, Dr. Catlin would prefer to see a well-designed study contrasting steroid use in School A with use in School B.

"If we're going to do testing," he continued, "we should find out what it's doing for us. The overall effect of testing seems to be to raise the level of knowledge and interest. In a sense, it's enforced learning." His message for coaches, school administrators and anyone involved with young people at risk is to pay attention to the issue.

"You cannot remain uninformed," he said.

The U.S./Russian Agreement

Drug testing on the international level, on the other hand, is viewed as a necessity, and there are signs that most countries want some type of universal agreement and sanctions. The U.S. Olympic Committee signed an agreement in June 1989 with the Soviet Union that would allow each nation to demand "short notice" — within 48 hours — testing of an athlete from the other country. Although the agreement only covers two countries, most drug experts expect the agreement to have an impact all over the world if the joint effort is successful.

"Once the program is going, athletes will have to clean up," Dr. Catlin said. "Then there will be pressure for everyone else to do it too."

Under the agreement, each country will provide a list of athletes who could be called in for short-notice testing by the other nation. The responsibility for submitting actual athlete names will rest with the national governing bodies of the individual sports. A positive test for steroids, drugs that mask steroids, or other prohibited drugs would ban the athlete from competition for two years. A second offense would result in a lifetime ban.

"We want to build up confidence in our athletes that the Soviets aren't using steroids while building up the Soviet's confidence that we aren't using them," said U.S. Olympic Committee president Robert Helmick.

For some time, Dr. Catlin has been working with Vitali Semenov, Ph.D., director of the IOC-approved laboratory in Moscow to standardize procedures and practices at the two facilities. Drug testing involves sophisticated and complicated technology, and testing methods may vary slightly from laboratory to laboratory, although a positive test in one IOC-approved laboratory should be a positive result in another. However, officials at UCLA and in Moscow are trying to make their testing exactly equivalent. The test substances will be formulated in precisely the same way, the same reagents will be used, and the lab methods will be identical. To accomplish this, there have been several exchanges of lab personnel, with the Russians spending time in California and the Americans going to the U.S.S.R. They have succeeded in getting the same configuration for instrumentation and developing joint computer programs, and, according to Dr. Catlin, they have also run test samples to compare data side by side.

"I can say that the progress is steady and that the willingness and cooperation are very high," he said. "The things that slow us down are that we don't have year-round exchanges, and communications between here and Moscow are not as good as they are with some other countries."

In reviewing how drug testing has affected sports so far, Dr. Catlin notes that it has been very effective in eliminating performance-enhancing drugs that must be taken during the event to work. Amphetamines, for instance, are easily detected, and their use has declined to almost zero in sports that have drug testing. They remain popular in sports that have a once-a-year announced test. Professional baseball players reportedly use them to stay alert during boring afternoons that may be punctuated by moments of stress and excitement. Athletes have reported that Syndocarb, a Soviet pharmaceutical drug that is supposed to have amphetamine-like properties, although it is different chemically, was used in Seoul by endurance athletes. The IOC laboratories are aware of this drug.

Anabolic steroids are quite a different story. No matter how good the laboratory is, it cannot find what is not there. Steroids are used in the training phase and, with the right timing, an athlete can use them before competition and drug testing. If any trace remains, however, it can be found.

Testing Procedures

Most competitors have very little idea what happens to the urine samples once they provide them, but the drug testing process actually begins right at the winner's stand.

At Olympic competitions, each sports venue has a doping control station. When a winner finishes his event, he is met by an escort who stays with him until the athlete reports to doping control (usually within 30 minutes). The escort is there to verify that the athlete does nothing to alter his physical status before he provides a urine specimen, and to protect him from possible sabotage by others. Because many athletes become dehydrated during their sports events, it is not uncommon for them to spend some amount of time in doping control. They may drink as many beverages as they wish, but these must come from sealed containers so that tampering cannot occur.

Remember Ben Johnson's claim that a "spiked drink" was responsible for his positive drug test? Johnson, of course, is the Canadian who won the 100-meter sprint at the 1988 Games in a blistering 9.79 seconds and then was disqualified when his drug test show he had taken stanozolol, a water-based oral anabolic steroid sold in Canada under the trade name Winstrol. Athletes who have positive drug tests almost always react by saying one of two things: A) "The laboratory made a mistake," or B) "Someone slipped me drugs when I wasn't looking." Johnson chose the B option and maintained his innocent victim posture until he testified under oath at the Canadian judicial hearing on drug use that he had been using anabolic steroids since 1981.

One difference between the national and Olympic drug testing programs and the one instituted at Homewood-Flossmoor High School is that Olympic Committee and NCAA rules require observation of the specimen collection. This has been a major stumbling block to testing programs, especially at the college level. Many athletes find observed voiding a distasteful procedure. A football player at Stanford University was asked how the procedure differed from simply using a urinal in a public bathroom and he replied that in a public bathroom, the man next to you is not there to watch you urinate but that the NCAA representative is there for no other purpose.

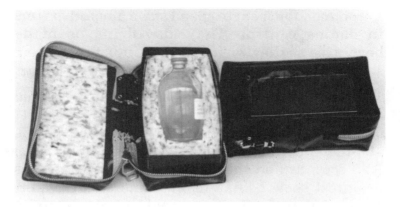

FIGURE 5-1. *One system used to maintain security of urine samples is the Envopak system developed by R.J. Brooks. After the observed urination, the athlete divides the sample into two numbered bottles like the one above. Each bottle is sealed and placed in the accompanying padded case, which is zipped and enclosed with a numbered plastic seal. The athlete verifies and annotates both the seal number and the sample number and then signs off on the doping control chain of custody sheet.*

Once the specimen is collected, it is divided into two parts, an A and B sample (Figure 5-1). The vials are closed, sealed, and marked by the athlete. Then a designated person must take charge, or custody, of the urine samples and that chain of custody must be documented from the testing station right to the laboratory. Otherwise, as Dr. Catlin has noted, he could not justify testing urine samples that "might have come from anywhere." When control is not maintained, there is a good chance samples will come from unlikely sources.

Inside the Laboratory

Once the sealed samples reach the laboratory, the B samples are refrigerated unopened and the A samples are opened and tested. The most common, and least expensive, type of initial screening is done by radioimmunoassay. These tests work on the basis of antibody response; that is, a substance in the test material will react with the class of drugs being sought. Immunoassays are used simply to screen large numbers of urine samples and they work well for broad classes of drugs, although they are not usually very specific.

Several different tests are run on each sample, screening for various classes of banned drugs. One might be for stimulants, another for beta-blockers and opiates, a third for caffeine, a fourth for anabolic steroids, and the fifth for diuretics.

The gold standard of drug detection is gas chromatography with mass spectroscopy (GC/MS) (Figure 5-2). This is used not only to confirm the presence of a banned drug but to identify it. Manfred Donicke, Ph.D., director of the IOC-approved laboratory in Cologne, West Germany, developed the test for anabolic steroids. Its introduction was the watershed event in drug testing. The previous test for anabolic steroids was not very reliable, and many users were not caught.

Dr. Donicke temporarily turned the tide in favor of the drug testers when he ran the laboratory that did the drug testing at the Pan American Games in Caracas, Venezuela, in 1983. Nineteen athletes were disqualified and scores more either withdrew from competition or purposefully did so poorly in competition that they did not win medals which would have caused them to be tested.

It would be nice to report that as a result of that competition, athletic drug use declined markedly. The actual result was that athletes who were using anabolic steroids switched from the

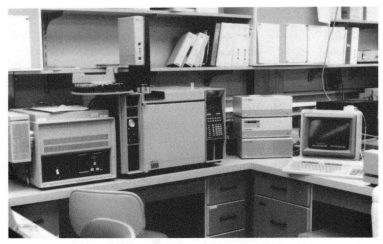

FIGURE 5-2. *This gas chromatography/mass spectrometry system (HP 5970B MSD) is used worldwide in urinalysis for steroids and other drugs.*

injected forms, which aren't as harmful to the liver, to the oral forms, which are more likely to cause liver and other problems but wash out of the system quicker, and to the esters of testosterone. Moreover, they also began looking for masking agents to hide their use of banned substances. Simple methods include adding a large quantity of water or some vinegar to the sample. Other drugs have been used to mask the presence of steroids.

One of the big stories of the 1987 Pan American Games was the revelation that some athletes were using probenecid, a drug not banned at the time, for masking purposes. Probenecid is one of a class of drugs known as uricosurics and it is used to treat gout or to reduce the rate of excretion of some other drugs such as antibiotics prescribed for sexually transmitted diseases. The IOC laboratories had no difficulty in detecting probenecid and it is on the banned list now.

An anabolic steroid test is expensive because the analysis takes a long time (eight to 12 hours), and the chemical preparation that must be done before analysis is lengthy and depends on very strict purity of reagents. When the mixture is placed in a gas chromatograph, it is separated into its components by passing through a column that permits some elements to pass through more quickly than others. Substances can be identified by the amount of time it takes to pass through the column. Next, the separated substance goes into the mass spectrometer detector. An electron beam causes the molecules to fragment into smaller pieces and the fragmented pieces form a pattern or "fingerprint."

By using gas chromatography/mass spectrometry, it is virtually impossible to misidentify a substance. Even so, when a sample contains a banned substance, the test is confirmed by using a different method of formulating the substance that goes into the gas chromatograph/mass spectrometer before it is reported as positive. Bear in mind that the laboratory usually is not looking for the drug itself but for metabolites. Each metabolite, and there may be many, has a distinctive pattern and building a library of them is time consuming and expensive. For instance, some drugs are sold only in Europe but the IOC-approved laboratories in the U.S. would still be expected to identify them. (The laboratories themselves get tested on a periodic basis by the IOC which sends them known, but unidentified, substances for testing.)

When an A sample is positive after the second time through the GC/MS, an official notification is made. For participants in the Olympic Games, notification goes to Prince Alexandre De Merode, chairman of the IOC Medical Commission and the person who keeps the list that matches athlete names with the identification numbers used by the laboratory. If it is an NCAA competition, the test results go first to the NCAA. When a sports governing body sponsors the testing, it get the results. The athlete also is notified that the test is positive.

When a sports governing body sponsors the testing, it gets the results. The athlete also is notified that the test is positive.

By Olympic or NCAA rules, the athlete and his coach or other representative may come to the laboratory and be present for the testing of the B sample, which up until now has remained sealed. If the athlete refuses to come or send a representative, the laboratory appoints someone not involved in the testing process to act in the athlete's interest. When an athlete makes a defense against a positive finding, he does it to the official sports governing body and not to the laboratory.

At Homewood-Flossmoor High School, parents of an athlete with a positive test may take a portion of the B sample to a laboratory of their choice for retesting. This might be feasible for substances other than anabolic steroids. However, the two urine samples designated for steroid testing each week go by air express to the Vanderbilt laboratory for testing there. Few commercial or hospital laboratories do steroid testing because of the expense of gathering and maintaining metabolic pattern "libraries" for the different steroids.

Beating the Tests

Despite testing, there will still be efforts to cheat, both with new drugs that become available, and by concealing evidence of drug taking. The fierceness of competition at the highest level has always stimulated athletes to look for something to give them a winning edge. The disturbing thing is that attitude seems to have filtered down to the lowest levels of competition so that the win/loss figures are seen as the only way to judge whether an activity was successful or worthwhile.

The fierceness of competition at the highest level has always stimulated athletes to look for something to give them a winning edge.

The Canadian hearings on the use of banned substances by athletes — an outgrowth of the Johnson scandal in Seoul — provided a good look at the way many athletes view drug use and the lengths they are prepared to go to avoid detection.

Four Canadian weight lifters headed for Korea got tripped up by an unexpected drug test before they left home. They testified at the Canadian hearings how they sweated it out in a Vancouver hotel room, discussing their dwindling options. They considered trying to bribe Sports Canada officials or staging a phony protest on some trumped-up matter so they could withdraw without being tested. Finally they hit upon the idea of obtaining "clean" urine specimens that they could inject into their own bladders.

"I was desperate," said David Bolduc, 23, one of those involved. "I was ready to do anything not to be caught."

Another of the group, Jacques Demers, who won a silver medal in weightlifting at the 1984 Olympics, testified that he was a steroid user then and he told Presiding Justice Charles Dubin, "If you wanted to be in the medal class, you had to use them."

The Canadian hearings also provided enlightening testimony about younger athletes who may be moving toward using banned drugs to enhance performance. Andrew Pipe, M.D., a cardiologist who chairs the National Advisory Council on Drug Abuse in Sport in Canada, told the court that a 15-year-old biathlete came to him at a university clinic to request beta blockers, a drug that slows the heart rate and which can help shooters maintain a steady hand. More disturbing, according to Dr. Pipe, was the fact that the youth told him his coach had suggested using this banned drug to advance in his sport. Beta blockers would be picked up easily by sports drug testing.

One of the most likely ways to get a false negative result (meaning the athlete is using the drug but was not detected) is to use a class of anabolic steroids called the esters of testosterone. As we said earlier, testosterone is a naturally occurring hormone so that any test must be based on determining when there is too much of a good thing. In the past, some athletes did escape detection by switching from anabolic steroids to testosterone a few weeks before a competition.

Then Dr. Donicke developed a test that uses the ratio of testosterone to epitestosterone, another naturally occurring hormone (which is the 17 epimer, or mirror three-dimensional image of testosterone, to be technical). In most normal people, the ratio is about 1 or 1.5, but it can vary. After looking at several thousand ratios, the IOC Medical Commission agreed to call it a positive result if the ratio of the total concentration of testosterone to epitestosterone in the urine was greater than 6 (T/E > 6/1 [6:1] = positive).

"I was desperate...I was ready to do anything not to be caught."

Penn State's Yesalis and R. Craig Kammerer, Ph.D., who was associate director of the UCLA drug laboratory during the 1984 Olympics, wrote an editorial in the February 4, 1990, issue of *The New York Times* calling the testosterone ratio "the Achilles' heel" of drug-testing programs. They claim that athletes who use low to moderate doses of testosterone, doses that Yesalis and Kammerer say exceed the amounts used by many strength athletes of the 1960s and early 1970s, could still get a clean drug test.

One of the first discussions of this potential loophole was at a National Institute of Drug Abuse (NIDA) consensus conference on steroids in 1989. Karl Friedl, Ph.D., said that while he was stationed at Madigan Army Medical Center in Tacoma, Washington, he was part of a research team that gave military volunteers either 100 or 300 mg testosterone or 19-nortestosterone (Deca-Durabolin) a week for six weeks as part of a study.

Urine samples from these volunteers were sent to a private laboratory to make sure the volunteers were not taking any other drugs. All Deca-Durabolin was detected, but both the low and high-dose testosterone samples were negative. Dr. Friedl telephoned the laboratory for confirmation. They rechecked their data and told him the ratio in the two men receiving the 300 mg dose of testosterone was 4.2:1, still well below the 6:1 figure. Although Friedl noted that the test involved a private laboratory and that only two of the test subjects received a high dose of testosterone, it remains an area of uncertainty. The average testosterone production in healthy males is approximately 6 mg a day, and administration of 100 mg a week of one of the long-acting esters such as the cypionate or enanthate will maintain normal physiological testosterone levels in adults.

This does not come as a surprise to the laboratory directors around the world, although they tend to think that each case where the ratio is unbalanced should be examined separately.

"If you look at the way testosterone is administered, it is quite possible to meter that administration so as not to test positive," says Robert Dugal, Ph.D. director of the IOC-approved laboratory in Montreal, Canada, and a member of the IOC Medical Commission. The question is, he adds, whether such a "metered dose" would have the desired effect.

"We know quite well that a value of 5:1, which would not even be reported out as positive, may represent someone who is using testosterone and getting away with it," says Dr. Catlin, adding that studies are underway to investigate how much normal variation there is in the ratio.

Keeping Quiet

Perhaps more disturbing than various testing loopholes are the reports that some sports governing bodies cover up drug use deliberately. Even the IOC has not been immune from such speculation.

During and after the 1988 Olympics, there were rumors that the IOC attempted to withhold news that Ben Johnson had failed his drug test in order not to cast a shadow over the event. The rumor gained currency when Jamie Astaphan, M.D., the physician who supplied Johnson with steroids, testified in Canada that he had been told that IOC President Juan Antonio Samaranch would have intervened to suppress the result had it not been leaked to a newspaper by someone at the Seoul laboratory.

Perhaps more disturbing than various loopholes are the reports that some sports governing bodies cover up drug use deliberately.

Samaranch dismissed the claims as "untruthful" and said a coverup would have been impossible, if for no other reason than that between 30 and 40 people knew about the positive result. At an IOC meeting in Colorado Springs in the fall of 1989, Arnold Beckett, Sc.D., director of the IOC-approved laboratory in London, said that suppression was never even mentioned. He added that Prince De Merode handed him a slip of paper with Johnson's name on it the night the commission was informed of the positive test and remarked that Dr. Beckett had been wrong to remark earlier that things were too quiet. Because of Johnson's "spiked drink" claim, the Medical Commission did take the somewhat unusual step of announcing that Johnson's steroid profile was inconsistent with one-time use.

It does seem likely that there have been instances where test results were suppressed by individual sports governing bodies. That may also be true in college and professional sports. Forest Tennant, M.D., the former NFL drug advisor, testified at a 1986 arbitration hearing that doctors and trainers representing half of the NFL's 28 franchises had told him that between five and 20 players on each of their teams were known drug users. Several college football programs have had major difficulty with team drug use in the recent past, with the University of Oklahoma at the top of the list. Anabolic steroid use there appears to have been just a minor item in a long catalogue of problems.

With many sports governing bodies moving to testing, it becomes important to look at the quality of the programs, realizing that anabolic steroid use will not disappear easily in many sports. The Athletics Congress, the national governing body of track and field, announced a year-round out-of-competition program in 1989. Under the program, the top 25 athletes in each event are subject to random testing any time during the year, with the name selection to be determined by computer. This could go a long way toward curbing the use of illicit performance-enhancing drugs by elite athletes in track and field if the program has realistic goals.

At the IOC meeting in Colorado Springs, there was an interchange between an official of a track group and Dr. Donicke, who presented a seminar on drug testing. The track official argued that anything lower than a 10:1 testosterone/epitestosterone ratio should be counted as normal, saying that this would protect men with extremely high levels of natural testosterone. However, in a later interview, Dr. Donicke said he had personally encountered only two athletes with a 10 ratio and that both had histories of previous steroid use. Another laboratory has had two athletes with apparently natural ratios above six, and it seems clear that more research on natural variations in the testosterone/epitestosterone ratio is needed.

Although substantial progress is being made toward international drug testing agreements, it seems apparent that educational efforts need to be stepped up, both with athletes and with their sports federations. At present, drug testing does not seem to be a practical solution to steroid abuse by younger athletes because of their numbers and because of the enormous cost. It might be worthwhile considering in areas of the country where steroid use is known to be heavy. All proposed drug testing programs should be scrutinized carefully to make sure they aren't by design or accident providing a cover for continued androgen use.

6

STEROIDS AND THE LAW

The legal issues that confront an anabolic steroid user can be divided into the following areas:
- What are the prospects of arrest and conviction on steroid-related charges?
- What effect will proposed federal legislation making steroids a controlled substance have?
- What are the legal responsibilities of coaches, trainers, and team physicians?
- Is drug testing legal, and for whom?

The federal government stepped up its efforts to prosecute anabolic steroid dealers and users in May 1986 by setting up a Task Force with the U.S. Department of Justice, the Food and Drug Administration, and the Federal Bureau of Investigation.

The first "name" athlete to be sent to prison after the formation of the interagency group was former British track star David Jenkins, who was sentenced to seven years and fined $75,000 in 1987. A California grand jury had returned a 110-count indictment against 34 individuals, including Jenkins, and two corporations. Jenkins entered a guilty plea in November 1987 for his part in a smuggling ring that prosecutors said dominated the U.S. black market for steroids at one time. The government prosecutors said Jenkins, holder of a silver medal from the 1972 Olympics, asked a Mexican citizen who owned a Tijuana pharmaceutical laboratory to manufacture counterfeit steroids there. The Mexican drugs bore fake labels that represented the steroids as being produced either by legitimate or fictitious drug companies.

One of the other 33 defendants indicted along with Jenkins estimated that $50,000 worth of steroids come across the border from Mexico every week and he remarked, "Even after all the busts, if I was a little kid in some hick town in Illinois, I could still get steroids."

"Even after all the busts, if I was a little kid in some hick town in Illinois, I could still get steroids."

Although he is probably right, some black market traders say the supply is tight as the government continues to pursue steroid smugglers and dealers (Figure 6-1). By the spring of 1990, there had been 125 legal actions on various steroid-related charges in 27 different federal districts. Approximately 85 people received jail sentences totaling 80 years on anabolic steroid-related charges. They have been fined $1.2 million and the government has seized $18 million worth of anabolic steroids, including counterfeit, diverted, and smuggled supplies.

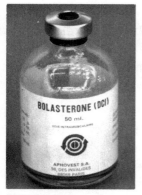 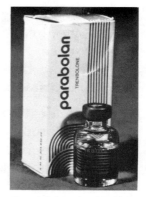

FIGURE 6-1. *Some steroids are produced by legitimate manufacturers in other countries and smuggled into the U.S. by individuals for sale to athletes. At left is Bolasterone, a counterfeit drug, and at right is Parabolan, a trade name for a real anabolic steroid, trenbolone acetate, used primarily in veterinary medicine but also in humans in other countries.*

Because the FDA has narrowed the approved types of anabolic steroids that can be marketed legitimately, a black market estimated to take in as much as $400 million a year continues to be a growth industry (Figure 6-2). (Until recently, the black market figure was $100 million, but federal law enforcement officials upgraded the amount last year). Sometimes agents find large caches of drugs when they arrest dealers. For example, at about the same time that Ben Johnson was confessing in Canada that he had been a steroid user for seven years before being caught by a drug test in Seoul, a former Mr. Universe, Luiz Batista Freitas, a Brazilian bodybuilder and weight lifter, entered a guilty plea in Los Angeles to keeping 10,000 anabolic steroid tablets on hand for distribution to other users.

Most pharmaceutical houses that manufacture steroids have stepped up their security efforts, and some steroids have actually been taken off the market, making it more difficult for black marketeers to obtain legally manufactured drugs. New sources have been created to serve the demand, and the government believes that many of the drugs now being sold could pose a health risk.

A clandestine steroid mail-order business in California promoted its products as East German drugs although they were actually manufactured in a secret laboratory in Fountain Valley, California. Because East German steroids have a reputation among athletes for being very good, the enterprising Californians had labels printed that read: Eigentum Der DDR-Versenden Gesetzlich Verboten, meaning property of the German Democratic Republic, export prohibited, and they sold them for $180 and up a bottle. Five people associated with that business were arrested, but not before the company openly advertised its products and received many telephone orders. The drugs were mailed to customers in packages marked Food Supplements.

A spokesman for the Justice Department said anabolic steroid offenses are "a high priority item" for the government. A major concern is that steroids are attractive to adolescents, a group particularly in need of protection because they are so frequently exploited by dealers. Many buy "drugs" that do not contain any active ingredients, and others buy substances that are unsterile and may have been manufactured under filthy conditions.

Even assuming that the drugs were diverted from US pharmaceutical houses and are of top quality, the claims for what they can do are almost always overstated by dealers. Naive teens of both sexes may believe the unbelievable, especially if

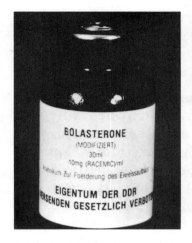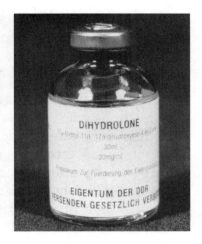

FIGURE 6-2. *The samples above are expensive counterfeit products that made hundreds of thousands of dollars for their producers, who have since been arrested and convicted for their activities. These products did not contain the substances specified on their labels but did contain some active steroids, although the amounts varied. Most of the counterfeit steroids produced and sold in the U.S. at this time include no active steroids, but as with veterinary drugs, they often contain adulterants which may cause immediate and serious health reactions. Counterfeit products cannot necessarily be distinguished by their labels, sizes, shapes, color, or consistency.*

advertising plays on their natural physical insecurities. While this insecurity is felt by both sexes, males tend to focus more on muscular development and strength. At a conference on health fraud in Kansas City, some of the most popular devices and potions identified were worthless muscle and breast developers and "miracle" diet pills. Most of these products were bought either by teenagers or young adults. Some of these same consumers see steroids as wonder drugs. They seem unaware that changes in muscle mass and strength are minimal or nonexistent without appropriate training programs and proper diet.

Even when younger steroid users are weight trained and using the drugs for the optimal effect, they can be harmed as much by buying black market products as by the steroids themselves.

It is only fair to say that young people are not the only ones who can be taken in by heavy hype of a product. Many seasoned athletes remember purchasing Bolasterone, a product that swept the country on the underground market, selling for as much as $275 a bottle. Bolasterone was supposed to be a super high-tech product from East Germany, one of the best steroids. By all accounts, however, it contained vegetable oil, a small amount of testosterone, and liquid aspirin.

Many (adolescents) buy "drugs" that do not contain any active ingredients, and others buy substances that are unsterile and may have been manufactured under filthy conditions.

In all likelihood, elite athletes are not obtaining their drugs from the same sources as younger users. David R. Lamb, Ph.D., a steroid expert at Ohio State University, says that most of the steroids used by athletes probably are not prescribed by physicians but are obtained directly from employees of pharmaceutical houses, from veterinarians, from pharmacists, or from other athletes who have obtained them while competing in foreign countries that don't have the prohibitions the U.S. does on dispensing these drugs. Some athletes do have assistance from physicians, and some drug experts think that physicians are probably the major source of steroids for top-level athletes.

Gateway Drugs?

Another concern on the part of government agencies is whether anabolic steroids are gateway drugs — that is, do they lead a user to try, and perhaps become addicted to, other illegal drugs. There are not enough data on which to base an informed opinion, although we do not believe that younger athletes who use steroids are likely to be the same people who are experimenting with marijuana and cocaine. As a group, steroid users are more interested in performance enhancement. This may not be the case with long-time users or with athletes whose wealth and fame have caused them to move in circles where recreational drugs may be used. Tony Fitton, a six-time British national power lifting champion, served a prison term for smuggling steroids into the U.S. from Tijuana during a period when he was a dealer. Fitton says that some athletes who blame their health problems on steroids were also using other drugs.

"I have known of quite a few strength athletes that have blamed heart problems on anabolic steroid use," he said. "The fact that these same athletes had an incorrigible propensity towards amphetamines and cocaine, they felt better left unmentioned. Anabolic steroids were a more socially acceptable excuse."

Certainly, a strong argument could be made that people willing to use illegal drugs are, at the very least, likely to use other substances that are illegal and illicit. These people are likely to be risk takers, rebellious, impulsive, and nonconforming.

We know that some anabolic steroid users take other drugs to counteract negative effects they get from steroids. We have almost no information on possible drug interactions that are capable of causing serious health problems by themselves. Heavy steroid users may use alcohol, marijuana, or tranquilizers to calm down, or barbiturates to sleep. Most experts agree that people who use heavy cycles probably increase their consumption of sedatives or hypnotics. They may also use specific other drugs to potentiate steroids or balance hormone levels. For example, Fitton claims that thyroid preparations are often used by bodybuilders and he believes they are more dangerous than steroids.

Heavy steroid users may use alcohol, marijuana, or tranquilizers to calm down, or barbiturates to sleep.

If anabolic steroids are gateway drugs, then users obviously increase their exposure to arrest. We believe that once a person accepts the principle of chemical performance enhancement, he is more likely to seek other drugs in that class. It also seems likely that users will turn to other drugs to blunt unwanted behavioral effects of steroids.

A Controlled Substance

Still another method to control anabolic steroids — adding them to the list of controlled substances — is being considered by Congress. Bills have been introduced in both the Senate and the House. A press conference on October 5, 1989, at which Congressman Mel Levine (D-Ca) announced the introduction of his legislation was a classic media event, with Canadian sprinter Ben Johnson making his first public appearance in the

U.S. since testifying in Canada about his own steroid use. Johnson received praised for his "courage in coming forward" to speak on behalf of the bill. However, Johnson's stance as a supporter of legislation to control steroids is suspect since he did not volunteer the information that he was a drug user, but rather was caught by a drug test. Moreover, he told reporters that had similar legislation been in effect in Canada, it would not have deterred him from using steroids.

American track star Carl Lewis, who has been outspoken about steroid use at the international level, attended the press conference. The irony inherent in the adulation our society gives to highly successful athletes was evident that day. Both Johnson and Lewis were photographed endlessly and asked many questions about steroids, while medical experts who had been asked to attend were shunted aside and largely ignored.

The proposed legislation has the support of some physicians and researchers, but other experts do not believe that anabolic steroids fit the criteria for classification as a controlled substance. The American Medical Association is on record as opposing, as a matter of principle, congressional rescheduling of drugs. The AMA believes this shortcut undermines the utility of the regular scheduling process. While Congress has the power to put any substances it wishes on the list, the normal process is for the Attorney General to act based on findings provided by the Secretary of the Department of Health and Human Services. The Attorney General must consider these factors before making a drug a controlled substance:

- The drug's actual or relative potential for abuse

- Scientific evidence of its pharmacological effects

- The state of current scientific knowledge about the drug

- Its history and current pattern of abuse

- The scope, duration, and significance of abuse

- The risk to public health

- Its capability to produce psychic or physiological dependence

- Whether the substance is an immediate precursor of a substance already on the list

Each drug that is classified in this manner is put on one of five schedules, with Schedule I drugs having the highest abuse potential and no accepted medical uses. Schedule I drugs include hallucinogens and heroin. Schedule II drugs have high abuse and dependence potential but they also have medical uses. Methamphetamine (known on the street as "speed") and cocaine are examples of Schedule II drugs. Schedule III drugs include stimulants, depressants, and narcotic drugs like codeine. Schedules IV and V drugs have the lowest abuse and dependence potentials. Both bills call for Schedule II status for steroids.

When a substance is controlled, special labels warning that it is illegal to transfer the drug must be used.Prescriptions cannot be automatically refilled. Manufacturers must keep close records of stocks and customer orders and amounts sold, and they must reregister every three years with the government.

In Washington, Levine told reporters, "We have a chance to stop steroids before they become as uncontrollable as cocaine." While that is a worthy goal, the argument weakens when we see that cocaine is a Schedule II substance and yet is widely available in the U.S. on the black market. Further, the Levine bill excepts veterinary steroids from scheduling although they are one of the largest sources of supply for the black market. The Levine bill establishes an interagency coordinating council that would develop a comprehensive national steroid strategy, and it also directs the Office for Substance Abuse Prevention to create programs for secondary schools. A number of states, beginning with Florida, Alabama, and California in the mid 1980s, have already reclassified steroids as controlled substances at the state level.

The heavy penalties for violating the Controlled Substances Act might discourage some potential dealers from trafficking in these drugs. Also, the act provides for forfeiture of property. A gym where steroids are available for sale could be seized by the government, just as boats are seized from cocaine drug runners. However, the Drug Abuse Act of 1988 also provides for forfeiture of property used to illegally manufacture or distribute drugs. It would undoubtedly be even more difficult to divert supplies from legitimate manufacturers. Also, it would allow the government to identify physicians who are prescribing anabolic steroids to athletes.

A few years ago, experts estimated that 20 percent of the steroids used by athletes were obtained by prescription (which is legal). This led Robert O. Voy, M.D., then the chief medical officer for the U.S. Olympic Committee in Colorado Springs, to observe that making steroids a controlled substance probably would have no effect on the black market. "What it would do is let us see which physicians are prescribing them, and for that reason alone, it might be a good idea," he commented. Dr. Voy now is medical director of the Las Vegas, Nevada, Institute of Physical Therapy.

Yet another concern voiced by the AMA about scheduling steroids is that the action could be used as a substitute for dealing with the problems in more effective ways. A spokesperson noted that merely reclassifying the drugs as Schedule II substances would not necessarily make money available for enforcement. The Drug Enforcement Administration already has its hands full dealing with cocaine and crack. We agree that this could be a valid concern. However, we don't know other methods of dealing with the problem that are guaranteed to be more effective. The AMA itself has not yet put forth any significant effort to develop such strategies.

Responsibilities of Others

The third area of legal interest deals with defining the responsibilities of others toward a steroid user. It is likely that the first people to suspect that someone is using anabolic steroids will be family members, friends, fellow athletes, coaches, and trainers. Because this behavior can be very secretive, it is also quite possible that no one will suspect until use is proven through drug testing.

When the first person to suspect steroid use is a team or private physician, his legal responsibility is based on the traditional physician/patient model. Drug abuse is considered to be an illness. Physicians are supposed to be able to diagnose illnesses and thus are legally obligated to attempt to confirm drug use and treat the patient.

It is likely that the first people to suspect that someone is using anabolic steroids will be family members, friends, fellow athletes, coaches, and trainers.

Because physicians have the greatest exposure, a side issue relating to their legal liability is of interest.Charles Kochakian, Ph.D., considered by many to be the father of steroid research, says that the frequent citing of adverse effects of steroids have served to encourage patients to sue physicians who may have prescribed steroids for legitimate medical conditions. A case he cited involved a Michigan physician whose patient had undergone surgery for an ulcer. After a long post-surgical period of unsuccessful conservative treatment, the doctor prescribed anabolic steroids. The patient was much improved after a month so the doctor gave her another injection of steroids. The next month, she reported that she continued to feel much better, but that her husband had advised her to sue because he had read that steroids were harmful. The legal responsibility of non-medical individuals, such as trainers or team managers, who might be in a position to know about athlete drug use has not been defined. There have been no known cases where an athlete has sued a coach or trainer for improperly encouraging steroid use.

Drug Testing

Drug testing is the fourth area where law and medicine interact. An excellent discussion of drug testing, indeed of all the legal considerations that arise from drug use, can be found in the book *Drugs and the Athlete* (Gary Wadler, M.D., and Brian Hainline, M.D., 1989, Philadelphia: F.A. Davis). The chapter titled "Legal Considerations" was written by H. Richard Beresford, M.D., J.D, a physician/attorney who is professor of neurology at Cornell University Medical College.

The International Olympic Committee has been in the drug testing business since the 1968 Olympic Winter Games in Grenoble, and the IOC program is so comprehensive that it serves as a model for some non-Olympic testing programs. IOC policies are used as general guidelines at many international sporting events, although organizing committees for those events often make modifications.

There is a movement for international agreement on sports drug testing and sanctions. The first permanent World Conference on Antidoping in Sport was held in June 1988 in Ottawa, Canada. At that time, participants agreed that everyone shares the responsibility for eliminating the use of drugs in sport, and a basic framework for agreement was established. Another meeting was held in Moscow in 1989, and standing committees are working out specifics for world accord on this subject. If such an agreement can be implemented (and many delegates believe that it can), and if the agreement includes out-of-competition testing, athletes really would meet on a "level playing field" at international meets. Meanwhile, the U.S. and the U.S.S.R. are trying to implement a bilateral agreement (see Chapter 5 on Drug Testing).

In addition to the Olympic programs, the national governing bodies of the more than 30 Olympic winter and summer sports may request testing and they may establish how often tests will be conducted.

The NCAA tests athletes for both performance-enhancing and recreational drugs, but does not require member institutions to administer testing programs during the year, although many do.

Outside the Olympic movement, where testing has been accepted as part of competition, athletes are most likely to be tested as part of a college program. The National Collegiate Athletic Association began a drug testing program in the fall of 1986 for participants in post-season competitions. The NCAA tests athletes for both performance-enhancing and recreational drugs, but does not require member institutions to administer testing programs during the year, although many do.

Many in the sports world, medicine, and law agree that a good case cannot be made for testing only athletes for recreational drugs because there is no evidence that they use these drugs any more or less than other college students or young adults.

Almost as soon as college drug testing began, the first legal actions were filed, and the first suits against the NCAA were lost. Stanford University diver Simone LeVant became the first athlete to successfully challenge the legality of the NCAA drug testing program. LeVant claimed that the drug tests were degrading, invaded her privacy, and constituted an illegal search. The American Civil Liberties Union (ACLU) opposes drug testing in principle and represented LeVant in the suit. Although she won an injunction against being tested, her case became moot when she failed to advance past the regional diving level. However, by 1987, the suit had been joined by two other Stanford athletes, Jennifer Hill, captain of the women's soccer team, and Barry McKeever, a football linebacker.

Santa Clara County Superior Court Judge Conrad Rushing eventually ruled that the NCAA program violates student-athletes' right to privacy as guaranteed by the California and U.S. constitutions. He also said the NCAA failed to demonstrate a compelling need to test student-athletes and that the program was too broad. For instance, although the NCAA tested 3,511 athletes in 1986 and 1987, only 34 students (including 31 football players) were declared ineligible for competition. The 34 positive tests included 26 where the drugs in question were anabolic steroids.

Meanwhile, up the Pacific coast at the University of Washington, another successful legal challenge to NCAA-mandated drug testing was mounted by Betsy O'Halloran, a freshman member of the track team. King County Superior Court Judge George Mattson ruled that the Washington plan violated state and federal constitutional guarantees of individual privacy rights against unreasonable search and seizure. The judge said the plan would only guarantee detection of a few addicted athletes and that this did not warrant the testing of hundreds of other athletes.

Now that some high schools are considering drug testing, it seems likely that some of these same issues will be heard in court again. Homewood-Flossmoor High School instituted a drug testing program for its athletes in 1989 after Head Football Coach John Wrenn told Athletic Director Kenneth Shultz that he suspected that some of his players were using drugs. When Coach Wrenn confronted them, they denied it. What about drug testing, he asked?

Before proceeding further, Shultz looked for a legal precedent that would cover high school drug testing. He found it in the Indiana case of Schaill vs Tippecanoe County. The 7th U.S. District Court of Appeals (the same federal district that Homewood-Flossmoor is in) had upheld drug testing of high school athletes, ruling that suspicionless searches are more likely to be permissible in circumstances where individuals have a diminished expectation of privacy. Because students athletes use communal dressing facilities and are required to undergo physical examination, the court held they met this criteria.

Shultz said the next move was deciding who among the 2,100 member student body to test. About 1,400 students participate in varsity sports during the year, 600 in fall sports, 300 in winter, and about 500 in the spring. The eventual decision was to randomly test 5 percent of athletes each week, for cocaine, marijuana, opiates, amphetamines, barbiturates, benzodiazepines, methadone, methqualone, phencyclidine, propoxyphene, alcohol, and anabolic steroids. Students must sign a consent form at the beginning of year and attend a training session before being allowed to participate in sports. Parents are notified of all results, within five days by mail if the test is negative. Students with positive tests are called within 48 hours by the student assistance coordinator. Parents and athlete must have an assessment interview with a chemical dependency counselor within 48 hours of notification unless they wish to have an independent test made (at their expense) on a portion of the B urine sample. The chemical dependency counselor makes a recommendation to the school on future athletic eligibility for any athlete with a positive test. Shultz says the program seeks to get help for athletes who need it, not just to punish them.

Although the Homewood-Flossmoor program appears to have broad-based community support, it remains to be seen whether high school drug testing is really feasible. However, the legal issues that come up will be much the same as those that have been tested in court at the college level. In general, the questions are: What are the privacy rights of athletes?, and, When can invasions of an athlete's privacy be justified?.

Dr. Beresford points out that the right to privacy is not an absolute guarantee of the Constitution, but rather an interpretation of the Constitution by the Court. The outer limits of this doctrine of privacy have not been absolutely defined and are still the subject of debate among legal scholars. However, most states have also enacted laws that protect individual privacy. This doesn't mean that drug users are free to claim that the Constitution protects their rights to do as they wish, just that they are protected against unreasonable searches and seizures, and against self incrimination.

Just as the IOC can bar athletes who won't agree to drug testing from competing, so can the NCAA or a high school. In professional sports, most athletes are covered by agreements negotiated by their unions or agents, and most of these call for a one-time announced drug test each year. However, the NFL has announced plans to test professional football players at least three times yearly, and other organizations may bargain with their players to get an increase in the number of drug tests.

Invading Privacy

The next legal point is how do we justify invasions of the privacy of athletes? Preventing drug users from taking unfair advantage and protecting athletes from drugs that may affect their ability to perform are two reasons with legal standing. Others are to protect the long-term health of athletes, and to identify those who may pose disciplinary problems or who are risking being permanently disabled.

Because anabolic steroids are supposed to be performance-enhancing drugs, the first legal question to be settled is whether they do actually enable an athlete to perform more skillfully. Only then can the question be asked whether the goal of drug-free competition is sufficient to justify coercive testing (testing that isn't undertake voluntarily). We may agree that anabolic steroids can enhance the performance of football players, but can we justify testing for them in sports where the value isn't clear, tennis, for example?

The process of drug testing is, itself open to legal scrutiny. Most athletes with positive tests claim that the laboratory made a mistake. The reliability of the testing method, the number of false positive and negative tests, the discrimination of the testing process for drugs of abuse are all areas of legal concern. At UCLA, more than 18,000 sports drug tests have been performed and, although the results have been challenged, not one has ever been overturned. It is very important for athletes and sports organizations to know that the testing process is reliable and that athletes will not be branded as drug users when they are not.

It is very important for athletes and sports organizations to know that the testing process is reliable and that athletes will not be branded as drug users when they are not.

One area of controversy in drug testing is whether to publicize the names of athletes with positive tests. Some sports medicine experts, including Dr. Voy, believe that publicizing the names serves as a strong deterrent.

"I am one who thinks that if we are going to solve the problem of drug use in sports, we have to expose those who cheat. I don't go along with aggregate figures. If an athlete has cheated the process, we need to make that public," says Dr. Voy.

Others like Don H. Catlin, M.D., director of the Olympic lab at UCLA, do not believe that the public has an absolute right to know this information.

"I think that, when the sports organization identifies a drug user through a test and imposes a sanction, that's the penalty," Dr. Catlin says. "I don't see the necessity of making a public announcement."

The NCAA itself does not publicize the names of athletes with positive drug tests; that is left to the individual colleges and universities. With big name athletes, it may be impossible to keep private the reason for nonparticipation. That was the case with Brian Bosworth, the Oklahoma linebacker who was barred from the 1987 Orange Bowl because of his steroid use. At the time, Bosworth railed at the NCAA and denied he was a steroid user. However, after becoming a professional football player, Bosworth wrote a book saying that anabolic steroids were popular drugs at Oklahoma.

The International Olympic Committee does release the names of athletes with positive drug tests, but Dr. Catlin notes that the U.S. Olympic Committee does not, and he adds: "As long as I am influential, they never will."

One last issue that interests legal scholars is whether athletes have any particular obligation to abstain from drugs. Other performers take various drugs without repercussions. A musician might take a drug to avert stage fright, a sedative so he could sleep before a performance, and an antihistamine to relieve a stuffy nose, while an athlete would be barred from taking any of them. The idea that sports represent an important social value and, therefore, must be protected is on somewhat shaky legal ground. It may be years before all the legal aspects of drug testing, including who shall be tested and under what conditions, have been defined so that both athletes and the courts are satisfied.

7

ETHICS

The January 8, 1990 issue of *Time* magazine included an article about how doctors are helping short children grow taller through injections of synthetic human growth hormone. These are not children doomed to be dwarfs because their pituitary glands do not produce this vital hormone, but children whose genetic makeup dictates shorter than average stature.

At first thought, this may seem a humanitarian act — albeit an expensive one at about $20,000 a year — helping short children become normal in height. However, if the door is opened to this type of drug use, we may quickly lose control of who goes through it.

The *Time* article quotes a professor of pediatrics at Yale University saying, "The question of who should and who shouldn't get growth-hormone therapy is a hornet's nest. The criteria are no longer clear." Not only is it true that the criteria are no longer clear, but how this drug is used has implications not only for how anabolic steroids may be used, but also for any currently available or yet to be developed drugs that enhance physical or mental abilities or performance.

The Food and Drug Administration approved the first genetically engineered human growth hormone in 1985 and the demand for it has grown steadily. (See Chapter 8 for a detailed discussion.) There have been thefts and diversions at both Genentech and Eli Lilly and Company, the two companies that manufacture the synthetic product.

One doctor told *Time* that as people realize they can control certain aspects of their appearance — orthodontia, face, nose, and breast reconstructions — they may also want to control height. The *Time* article told how an author of how-to-succeed-in-business books asked for human growth hormone therapy for his son saying, "I'd rather my son be 5 feet 10 inches and a graduate of New York University's business school than 5 feet 6 inches and a Harvard Business School graduate. These extra four inches in height make much more difference in terms of success in a business career than any paper qualifications you have."

It takes no great leap of imagination to envision how much more successful some athletes could be if they were taller or bigger. How many athletically talented high school kids have been cut from basketball teams or relegated to the "B" squad simply because of height? Doug Flutie had a brilliant career as a college football player, winning the Heismann Trophy, but his NFL career has been hampered by the fact that at about 5 feet, 8 inches, he is short for a quarterback.

The ethical question in all of this is, of course: Do we have the right to alter our physical (or mental) makeup in order to compete more successfully in sports or other areas of life? If we allow physical alterations to occur for business purposes — a frequent happenstance in the entertainment business — or because we desire to look different, can society ethically deny the same right to athletes? At a basic level, this point is part of the larger question of whether life belongs to the individual or to society.

Just Another Tool

Many athletes have dealt with the issue of whether they have the right to alter physical makeup to their own satisfaction, which is why most who have taken performance-enhancing drugs feel no shame or embarrassment about it. They view performance-enhancing drugs as simply another tool, along with good nutrition, food supplements, and scientific physical training methods, to be used to achieve a goal. There are physicians who would agree. Plenty of coaches and trainers share this view.

The ethical question in all this, of course: Do we have the right to alter our physical (or mental) makeup in order to compete more successfully in sports and other areas of life?

Frederick Hatfield, Ph.D., a former power lifter who was once the scientific editor of *Muscle & Fitness* expressed this point of view quite well when he wrote: "I believe that drugs have been, are and will continue to be an important source of man's salvation. I also believe that there can be no nobler use for drugs than improving man's performance capabilities. Society demands bigger, faster, and stronger athletes. The sacrosanctity of the sports arena, however, has been a hindrance to meeting this demand." (Like some other scientists who originally saw no harm in athlete use of anabolic steroids, Dr. Hatfield has changed his views and now is outspoken in his opposition to the use of steroid and other performance-enhancing drugs on both health and ethical grounds.)

If society accepts the validity of his original perspective, as many in sports still do, then there is no problem with an athlete using anabolic steroids to enhance performance, or indeed, anything else.

They view performance-enhancing drugs as simply another tool, along with good nutrition, food supplements, and scientific physical training methods, to be used to achieve a goal.

An 1989 article in *Sports Illustrated* by Rick Telander told how Tony Mandarich, an outstanding college lineman who was drafted by the Green Bay Packers, prepared for his daily workout by ingesting a large amount of caffeine. Telander also noted that there have been rumors, denied by Mandarich, that he uses steroids. Whether or not Mandarich uses steroids, he obviously accepts the principle of chemical performance enhancement if his caffeine intake is actually as high as reported. Although caffeine is a legal drug, it is nonetheless a drug and it can cause nervousness, irritability, insomnia, a rise in blood pressure, and changes in heart rate and rhythm. It also can cause delirium, seizures, coma, and death in extreme cases. It is on the International Olympic Committee banned drug list in high amounts (12 ug/ml). The point in all this is that if you accept the use of drugs for performance enhancement of any kind, what difference does it make which drug you use?

Many non-athletes also rely on caffeine to get them going in the morning and keep them going at night. Caffeine is a widely used legal drug, and few people ever even think of it as a drug at all.

At the other extreme of the performance enhancement spectrum is a report of the natural manipulation of hormones so repugnant that it makes drug use pale by comparison. John Hoberman, Ph.D., and Terry Todd, Ph.D., both faculty members at the University of Texas, Austin, have called to our attention to a rare practice called "pregnancy doping." According to Dr. Hoberman and Dr. Todd, the big topic of conversation at a gynecological meeting in France in 1988 was female athletes who became pregnant to benefit from the hormonal changes, then had abortions before the pregnancies advanced enough to hurt their training. Presumably there were no reports of such a corrupt practice on the meeting agenda. However, the credibility of the reports have been bolstered, Dr. Hoberman and Dr. Todd say, by the successful sports performances of women athletes after they became mothers.

Several women athletes who have borne children discovered that their sports performances actually improved. This may have been the stimulus for other women to try to obtain the benefits without actually delivering children. This is, of course, an extreme example of deliberate manipulation of natural hormones in an immoral way. Many would argue that it is not in the same class as taking synthetic hormones.

Differences of Opinion

The ethics of taking hormones that come from outside the body to enhance sports performance have been weighed by many intellectuals who have sometimes reached different conclusions. Norman Frost, M.D., a professor of pediatrics and director of the program in medical ethics at the University of Wisconsin School of Medicine, noted in 1983 that many athletes seek advantages through special diets, rigorous training, outstanding coaching, and meditation. He said that using steroids could be compared to using special exercise machines or eating high protein meals, both of which help an athlete build muscle tissue. Taking steroids, he continued, cannot be distinguished from other "tortures, deprivations, and risks" to which athletes subject themselves to achieve success, and he asserted that athletes who find the costs excessive are free to withdraw from that lifestyle.

Another point of view — one with strong support from most sports medicine experts and the authors — has been put forward by Thomas H. Murray, Ph.D., director of the Center for Biomedical Ethics at the School of Medicine at Case Western Reserve University in Cleveland. The use of performance-enhancing drugs, he says, "is a form of cheating, counter to the quest for physical excellence that sport is supposed to honor. We keep coming back to the ideal of excellence," he has said, "and the purpose of sport as the encouragement and reward of excellence. If this is true, as I believe it is, then drugs and other performance aids should be banned because they do not reflect the forms of human excellence that sport is intended to honor."

In Dr. Murray's view, using drugs distorts the nature of sport, and rewards differences among competitors — such as the willingness to risk good health — that are not among the forms of excellence that we believe are important and relevant to the sport.

The use of performance-enhancing drugs "is a form of cheating, counter to the quest for physical excellence that sport is supposed to honor."

He disagrees with Dr. Frost who has said concern about athletic use of steroids is paternalistic and disingenuous, by saying there is nothing wrong with attempting to reduce any risks that are not part of the intrinsic nature of the sport. In that sense, many sports do take steps to reduce the risk of injury. Football rules prohibit grinding the quarterback into the turf after he has gotten rid of the ball, in an effort to protect these key players from unnecessary harm. Are those rules paternalistic?

The Hastings (on Hudson, N.Y.) Center conducted a two-year dialogue from 1979 to 1981 on the place of drugs in American society that looked at moral, legal, and social viewpoints. The main points of that dialogue are:

- That society's response to nontherapeutic drug use has been irrational and inconsistent;

- That attempts at control have been clumsy and ill-informed; and

- That many complex moral values are entwined in the debate which cannot be reduced to a simple conflict between individual liberty and state paternalism.

Dr. Murray, who serves on the Committee on Substance Abuse, Research, and Education of the U.S. Olympic Committee, believes society is wrong to tolerate a system where only those who cheat succeed.

Although many athletes and coaches who have condoned or silently tolerated the use of anabolic steroids because they believe their use "evens the competition" or "levels the playing field," there are those who fear that the use of drugs for performance enhancement affects society in general and that the effect is negative and may be permanent.

Terrible Experiments

There can be no doubt that the effects of some drug experiments, in which athletes were, in effect, guinea pigs for their doctors, coaches, or handlers, have had negative and permanent results.

Birgit Dressel, a 26-year-old West German heptathlete (the heptathlon, in which women compete in seven track and field events, corresponds to the men's decathlon), died in April 1987 under mysterious circumstances. The German newsweekly, *Der Spiegel,* published excerpts of a report by a government investigative committee. Dr. Hoberman and Dr. Todd call the case "one of the ugliest chapters in the recorded history of sports medicine." Like many other top West German athletes, Dressel saw a particular doctor, a radiologist with an interest in sports. According to the article, from the time Dressel was 20 until her death, this doctor injected her at least 400 times with dozens of substances, not counting injections and pills she gave herself at home. One of the last injections she was given was a gold compound. After she died in agony, an autopsy revealed that the sheer number of foreign substances in her body, including various forms of anabolic steroids, made it impossible to determine the exact cause of death.

Competing in elite sports is in itself a stress that disrupts the reproductive systems of many female athletes, so that they pay a physical price for their athletic success under the best of circumstances. Puberty may be delayed in girls, and the menstrual cycle may cease in young women, putting them at risk of bone loss. Temporary infertility is likely, particularly when women take anabolic steroids, and there have also been reports of birth defects in the offspring of women athletes with a history of steroid use. Murray reports that he has heard of two women who were world champions in the 1970s who appeared to age with stunning rapidity, and that their competitors strongly suspect that steroids were a major factor.

As a society can we really be concerned about the ultimate welfare of women like Birgit Dressel if we subscribe to the ethics of a Swedish strength coach who said in 1984, "Our ethical and moral rules have maintained that one must not administer anything to the body. But I view the hormonal substances as a progressive development comparable to the use of fiberglass poles by vaulters."

Then we must ask: What is the end point of such development? In 1985, the president of the Federal Republic of Germany, Richard von Weizsacker, told the West Germany National Olympic Committee that the temptation to treat the human body as if it were a machine conflicts with our most basic ideas of what a human should be. He believes sport will be able to preserve its humanizing influence and contributions to human dignity only by resisting pressure to use chemical or genetic manipulations to achieve results.

Those remarks were reported by Dr. Hoberman, who is an associate professor of Germanic languages, in a speech at a symposium sponsored by the University of Texas Ethics Lecture Series. Dr. Hoberman said that high-performance sport "has become an exercise in human engineering that aims at producing not simply an athletic type, but a human type as well."

...sport will be able to preserve its humanizing influence and contributions to human dignity only by resisting the pressure to use chemical or genetic manipulations to achieve results.

He is concerned that the increasingly high-tech nature of sports contains, and in some ways conceals, an agenda for human development for which high-performance athletes serve as ideal models. Moreover, he concludes "this anthropological agenda is a sinister one that transcends, even as it includes, cultivation of certain body types for sportive purposes."

Dr. Hoberman noted that the bodies of many high-performance athletes have become, quite literally, laboratory specimens; that structure and potential can be measured in precise terms. Already, we have the body composition analyzer which describes the body in terms of water, fat, and other tissues; the force platform that measures biomechanical force; and the digitizer, a computerized device that translates athletic movements into a moving stick figure on a computer screen so that the composite parts can be analyzed separately. Dr. Hoberman says these procedures are a dimension of sport that the public knows little about but probably would not find objectionable since they measure the organism rather than change it.

"This anthropological agenda is a sinister one that transcends, even as it includes, cultivation of certain body types for sportive purposes."

However, the step from measurement to change is a small one. If a football player suffers a sprain, is it all right to tape it and give him an injection to deaden the pain so he can play or does that constitute performance enhancement? If it is acceptable for an athlete to use drugs to perform a feat that would otherwise be impossible, then what is wrong with taking the next step of using drugs to enhance the performance?

Dr. Hoberman believes these next years will continue to be difficult ones for coaches primarily because they face strong contradictory demands. On the one hand, they are expected to improve performance while, on the other, they are also expected to represent traditional values. This is no theoretical dilemma, by any means.

Most people would agree that the University of Oklahoma football program, where some young athletes ended up being arrested for such diverse felonies as selling cocaine and gang rape, spiraled out of control because the pressure to win led to a mindset that it was acceptable to do anything so long as the team stayed on top. Brian Bosworth, an Oklahoma player who was one of the 27 college football players (from at least seven universities) who tested positive for anabolic steroids in 1986 and, thus, were not permitted by NCAA rules to participate in postseason play, was highly critical of the NCAA for the drug testing.

If it is acceptable for an athlete to use drugs to perform a feat that would otherwise be impossible, then what is wrong with taking the next step of using drugs to enhance performance?

"Steroids are a legal drug," he said. "I'll continue to fight against the abuse of drugs — recreational drugs that are destroying society. Steroids aren't destroying society."

The latter statement is surely open to question. Bosworth claimed when he was barred from playing in the Orange Bowl that he really wasn't a steroid user anyway; he only took them because they were prescribed by a doctor to help heal an injury. However, he told a different story about drug use at Oklahoma in his autobiography, claiming that all drugs were available and used. In any event, the free-wheeling, above-the-law attitude of Oklahoma players provided concrete proof of the observation by Swiss psychiatrist Carl Jung that we become what we do. After the chaotic situation at Oklahoma eventually caused the resignation of Football Coach Barry Switzer, the new coach instituted strict rules of behavior for the players.

Looking for Consensus

In truth, steroids are a fact of life in many college AND high school football programs, and with other genetically engineered drugs on the horizon, we still have not reached a consensus ethical position on steroids.

William N. Taylor, M.D., says time is running out. In his book, *Hormonal Manipulation: A New Era of Monstrous Athletes*, Dr. Taylor writes:

"Medical scientists have progressed to a point at which they can identify, isolate, and subsequently synthesize many of the major hormones of the body so quickly that even the scientists cannot begin to study the effects of these hormones on humans prior to their release on mankind....And the sports medicine world is not even yet sure how to handle the anabolic steroid issue which is over a decade old! We simply do not have the luxury of a decade of time to determine which avenues mankind will take along the paths of the continuing saga of hormonal manipulation of humans."

Dr. Murray has said that any argument for prohibiting or restricting drug use by Olympic athletes must contend with a powerful defense based on our concept of individual liberty.Our tradition of personal liberty holds that we have the right to pursue whatever plans we have and to take risks if we wish and, within broad limits, to do with our bodies what we wish. As Dr. Murray notes, many recreational and occupational pursuits afford much more risk than taking steroids: mountain-climbing, hang-gliding, coal-mining, and high-steel construction work. Dr. Murray makes the base of his argument against steroids the fact that their use is coercive.

"We simply do not have the luxury of a decade of time to determine which avenues mankind will take along the paths of the continuing saga of hormonal manipulation of humans."

"Olympic and professional sport, as a social institution, is an intensely competitive endeavor, and there is tremendous pressure to seek a competitive advantage," he said. "If some athletes are believed to have found something that gives them an edge, other athletes will feel pressed to do the same, or leave the competition. Unquestionably, coerciveness operates in the case of performance-enhancing drugs and sport."

Dr. Murray notes that all sports have rules and the person who wins at a sport does so because he performs better than any of the competitors within the rules. If you take a 10-yard head start in a race or put 12 football players on the field instead of 11, you break the rules of the sport. Changing the rules may alter performance, Dr. Murray argues, but not necessarily the standing of the competitors. If everyone uses a 12-pound shot instead of the regulation 16-pound one, everyone will throw it farther, but the best at 16 pounds will probably also be the best at 12. If we give all shot-putters 10 mg of Dianabol a day, he continues, you might produce a similar situation, but you have greatly increased the risk of competition for the athlete.

"A willingness to take health risks by consuming large quantities of steroids is not one of the desired, legitimate differences among competitors," Dr. Murray observes.

We could do what has been advocated for recreational drugs. Simply make them legal and let those who wish to use drugs use them. No, says Dr. Murray, that won't work either.

"A willingness to take health risks by consuming large quantities of steroids is not one of the desired, legitimate differences among competitors."

"Changes that affirmatively tempt athletes to take the maximum health risk are the worst," he says. "Lifting the ban on performance-enhancing drugs would encourage just that sort of brinkmanship."

The Canadian Hearings

While the athlete is the person who actually takes the drug and, thus, the biggest health risk, athletes are often so controlled by coaches, personal trainers, or sports doctors or psychologists that they resemble a product produced by a group rather than individual athletes. The man behind Canadian sprinter Ben Johnson was his coach, Charlie Francis, who told Johnson he would not be able to compete at the world level without using steroids. At the Canadian judicial hearings on the use of drugs in sports, Francis testified under oath how he told Johnson "the facts of life" about world competition in 1981.

"He could decide either he wanted to participate at the highest levels in sport or not," said Francis. "He could set up his starting blocks on the same line as all the other competitors in international competition, or set them up a metre behind them." '

The man behind Canadian sprinter Ben Johnson was his coach, Charlie Francis, who told Johnson he would not be able to compete at the world level without using steroids.

Francis said repeatedly that his Number 1 concern was the well-being of his athletes and that he did not believe there were harmful side effects from steroids at the low doses and regulated cycles in which his athletes used them. He seemed surprised when Johnson's lawyer asked him if he was aware that Johnson's personal physician had detected a mild swelling in the sprinter's left breast in the fall of 1987 (at that time, Johnson told his doctor that he did not use steroids).

During his testimony, Coach Francis charged that all world-class track athletes use banned drugs, and he said that some countries, including the U.S., go to great lengths to protect them from being detected. Francis claimed that before the 1984 Olympic Games in Los Angeles, the U.S. had an informal policy approved by the U.S. Olympic Committee (which denies it) that athletes could go in for regular tests to find out how long it took their systems to clear the drugs they used, a practice one drug laboratory head calls "peek-a-boo tests."

What the U.S. Olympic Committee actually did was conduct drug testing at a number of sports events in the early 1980s with no penalties for positive results. The idea was to educate athletes about drugs and drug testing before testing became a required part of U.S. sports events. Robert O. Voy, M.D., then chief medical officer for the U.S. Olympic Committee, has said that about half the athletes had positive tests, and that he now believes the project was ill-advised in that it allowed some athletes time to figure out how to beat the tests rather than conform to the policy.

The Canadian hearings may have a very positive on sports eventually, because they stripped away hypocrisy and exposed ethical issues. After Johnson was disqualified in Seoul and lost his 9.79 second world record in the 100-meter sprint, the Canadian government appointed a commission to investigate the country's athletes. Ontario Associate Chief Justice Charles Dubin, head of the commission, has said: "I think it is important to consider whether there are pressures being placed on our young men and women athletes to tempt them to cheat. Have we, as Canadians, lost track of what athletic competition is all about?"

In fact, Canada has taken the lead in promoting fair competition and exposing unethical practices. Having a Canadian type of hearing in the U.S. would not be possible because our athletes do not receive government financial support, and sports are not government-regulated, as is the case in Canada.

However, another area of ethical strain that can be expected to continue and perhaps increase for several years in this country and some others is between athletes and the national sports governing bodies that set the rules for competition and the drug-testing procedures. There have been instances where these procedures have been manipulated in order for athletes to participate and win while still giving the appearance of complying with the idea of a drug-free event.

Richard Pound, a Montreal, Canada, attorney who is a vice president of the International Olympic Committee, testified at the Canadian sports hearings that he believes the International Amateur Athletic Federation manipulated drug tests in at least one championship competition, the 1983 world championship in Helsinki, Finland. There have been rumors in the U.S. for the last seven years that one of the top U.S. track stars tested positive in Helsinki. Although the IOC-approved drug testing laboratories do excellent work, their findings are reported to sports governing federations who decide what action to take. Obviously, it would be a major ethical violation for a federation to conceal positive drug tests or manipulate testing results. Another legitimate conclusion from such conduct would be that concealment perpetuates drug use.

A Bigger Issue

The ethical issues of drugs in sports are far broader than simply those that revolve around athletes taking anabolic steroids. How they get those drugs and whether they are pressured to use them, so that they never really give "informed consent," is also an issue.

A separate issue is the ethics of physicians who administer drugs that may have deleterious effects on health, not really at the urging of athletes but in an attempt to make them into super specimens. Then there are "advisors" in gyms, usually people who are relying on a body of anecdotal evidence that has no basis in scientific fact when they assure young users that anabolic steroids will cause them no harm. What ethical responsibility do they bear? In the larger cities, personal trainers are becoming increasingly popular. These individuals may provide work-out techniques, diets, and nutritional supplements for their clients. Sometimes they recommend and provide drugs. Some of these personal trainers may be steroid users themselves and they may exert a strong influence on their clients.

"I want to spit on myself. Not because of the way I look, but because I let it happen to myself."

Still another ethical consideration is what happens to the athlete when the competition finally is finished forever? A Dutch study of women who participated in World, European, and Olympic championships over a 10-year period concluded that these women had a number of psychological problems, drug dependencies, and suicidal impulses. Dr. Hoberman says the worst cases may involve female athletes who have let male coaches persuade them to take drugs.

"I want to spit on myself," Dr. Hoberman quoted one of them as saying. "Not because of the way I look, but because I let it happen to myself."

In a 1990 article on women's bodybuilding, author Laura Dayton says that steroids have caused the sport to become perverted from the original intent of providing a new forum for appreciation of the female form. She notes that the drugs are basically the same hormonal therapy a transsexual would use to change secondary sex characteristics to those of a man.

"I have personally known women bodybuilding competitors who have had to tape their steroid-enlarged clitoris down to keep the bulge from showing during competition," Dayton wrote. "I know several who wear wigs because steroids have caused their hairline to drastically recede. Other friends have developed deep bass voices."

Women who take steroids are much more likely than men to have long-lasting negative effects, but men are not immune. Those individuals who help athletes and others make the decision to try drugs, those who supply them, those who assure users they won't be harmed, and those who experiment with drugs are helping to create a situation where the quest for excellence becomes so distorted and perverse it becomes merely an exercise in creative biochemistry.

It is clear that we need some national consensus on what constitutes ethical conduct. Dr. Hoberman says that if we take technological advances to the conceivable limit, we may end up developing a highly efficient, machine-like being who will be naturally cruel and combative (because those qualities give a competitive edge). Is that where we want to go?

8

PERFORMANCE ENHANCEMENT

Enhancing sports performance covers a lot of territory. It includes more than banned drugs. A good night's sleep enhances performance. Good nutrition, physical training programs, proper training technique — all of these strongly affect the quality of sports performance. Proper mental preparation is probably the single most important factor in athletic success, and sports psychology is a fast growing field. When a professional athlete has a bad day, most often the psychological components of sports performance are responsible. At the elite level, very slight differences in psychological preparedness can translate into success or failure.

What we think of as the dark side of performance enhancement is cheating to gain an advantage over your opponent. It is Rosie Ruiz running triumphantly across the finish line in the Boston Marathon after taking the subway most of the way. Everybody recognizes this behavior for what it is — cheating. Sometimes people don't recognize or accept the use of anabolic steroids, other banned substances, or blood doping as cheating. Adopting these methods is far more subtle than simply giving yourself a whopping head start in a race. However, using chemicals that may give a significant edge, even though they carry a significant risk to health along with any benefits, is still against the rules. Moreover, the fact that a top athlete is willing to take this risk forces others who want to compete to consider taking the same risks. Will the outcome of future sports events be decided by which side has the best chemists and whose athletes are willing to take the biggest risks (Figure 8-1)?

Both right and wrong ways to enhance sports performance will be considered in this chapter. There are other banned drugs and questionable practices besides those we cover in this limited space. We have chosen not to discuss any of the so-called recreational drugs — cocaine, marijuana, alcohol — although they clearly have effects on athletic performance.We recommend the excellent book, *Drugs and the Athlete*, by Gary Wadler, M.D., and Brian Hainline, M.D., (1989 F.A. Davis, Philadelphia) for a full discussion of all the drugs that can affect sports performance.

Banned Drugs

Many drugs besides anabolic steroids are on the list of drugs that are banned by the International Olympic Committee (IOC) or the National Collegiate Athletic Association (NCAA) because of their potential to enhance athletic performance. Like many physicians, we believe the list has be-

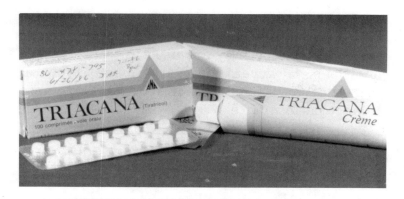

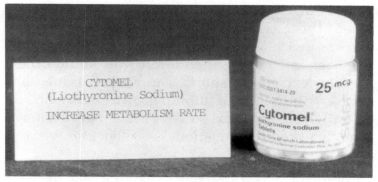

FIGURE 8-1. The non-steroid substances above are used by some athletes to enhance appearance. (Top) Triatricol is chemically related to thyroid hormones. Manufactured in France, where it is used in the treatment of obesity, it is one of many products smuggled into the U.S. by and/or for bodybuilders. The oral form is used to stimulate metabolism in an effort to reduce body fat, and in some cases, the metabolism and excretion of anabolic steroids in individuals who are subject to urinalysis for steroids. The cream is used by some prior to physique competitions in the belief that it assists in eliminating fluid from and tightening the skin. (Bottom) Liothyronine sodium (marketed as Cytomel and numerous other trade names) is a fast-acting, high-potency thyroid hormone used by some athletes to stimulate metabolism and promote loss of body fat. Medical data do not support the efficacy of these products in obesity treatment unless there is an underlying thyroid function disorder. A number of health risks are associated with the use of these and other metabolic stimulants. Serious reactions may occur with high doses and, even in modest doses, normal thyroid function may be reduced and otherwise disturbed for significant periods after use is terminated.

come too long (43 pages of fine print) and includes some drugs that should be allowed (in therapeutic amounts) because they are used to treat medical conditions. However, there are several types of drugs that serve no purpose in sports other than to enhance performance.

Will the outcome of future sports events be decided by which side has the best chemists?

HUMAN GROWTH HORMONE (hGH) is one of these (Figure 8-2). This drug went on the market in 1985 and, as we noted in Chapter 7, it has been used to treat children who would otherwise be extremely short. The ethical issue that arises with the use of human growth hormone has actually come to pass in that some parents have already asked the question, "Too short for what?"

Most physicians view drugs as a tool to return patients to a state of normality. Obviously, if a pediatrician has a child whose pituitary gland doesn't secrete growth hormone, he can help that patient achieve a state of near normality by giving him growth hormone. Some people, on the other hand, are genetically destined to be shorter than average just as others are destined to be taller, or thinner, or heavier than average. The question of what is normal then becomes very significant.

We don't know how many athletes are using or have used synthetic growth hormone, although the number is nowhere near that of anabolic steroid users for several reasons, one being that its purported effects on performance are not as clear. Price is another deterrent to the use of hGH, as is the fact that it must be kept refrigerated. Obtaining enough human growth hormone to produce an ergogenic effect (this is, aid performance) could cost as much as $10,000 a year, according to one expert, while another says an eight-week supply would probably run between $1,000 and $1,500.

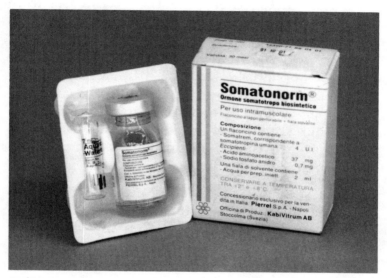

FIGURE 8-2. *Somatonorm is one brand of human growth (or somatotrophic) hormone. It is a protein hormone that promotes the growth of all body tissues, stimulates protein anabolism, and affects mineral metabolism. It is available in a "natural" form, extracted from the pituitary glands of cadavers, and as a genetically engineered, biosynthetic product. When administered to individuals whose ephiphyses are closed, it causes acromegaly in which facial features become course and the hands and feet become enlarged. Antibodies are formed in some patients; there is a diabetogenic effect on carbohydrate metabolism, and hypothyroidism may develop during treatment. There appears to be a slight increase in risk of leukemia in hormone-deficient patients treated with growth hormone that may be magnified by long-term administration. The health repercussions of uncontrolled growth hormone use by athletes are not known. Counterfeit products containing no active ingredients are avaiable on and have been confiscated from the black market.*

What do athletes think it will do for them? They believe it will give them many of the same benefits as they get with anabolic steroids, an increase in lean muscle mass and strength, a decrease in body fat, and an increase in bone growth. Many athletes believe hGH potentiates the action of steroids, so they get a greater effect by taking them together than they could get from taking either drug alone. These are all desirable effects to drug users, but no one is certain whether the currently recommended doses would allow the effects to be realized. Don H. Catlin, M.D., director of the IOC-approved drug testing laboratory at UCLA, says, "Every time I read anything about the doses that are recommended to athletes, they are nothing more than homeopathic," that is, they aren't high enough to bring about physiological changes.

There are serious doubts about the purity and potency of the supply of hGH on the U.S. black market. Bob Goldman, D.O., founder of the High Technology Fitness Research Institute in Chicago, says that his sources tell him athletes often do not get what they pay for. "The business is a great source of income for sellers on the black market," he says. "They're getting true drug prices for solutions that are just salt water."

His comments are seconded by Mauro di-Pasquale, M.D., a sports drug expert in Canada, who reports that smuggling real hGH in from other countries is difficult because of the refrigeration issue. "Even if it is viable hormone to begin with, it often isn't by the time the athlete takes it," he says.

Interestingly enough, human growth hormone is secreted over the whole of a person's life, although we really don't know the exact function of hGH in adults. John R. Sutton, M.D., a Canadian physician who is a former president of the American College of Sports Medicine, has explained that a wide variety of stimuli affect human growth hormone which is secreted by the pituitary and released in a pulsating fashion. Exercise, sleep, and the intake of certain foods or drugs affect release, and the strength of the response to hGH secretion varies with age, sex, and the stage of physical maturity.

The (hGH) business is a great source of income for sellers on the black market. They're getting true drug prices for solutions that are just salt water.

As early as the 1930s, breeders noted that animals that were given a crude extract made of pituitary glands of other animals of their own species had a marked increase in muscle mass and a decrease in body fat. They also grew faster. Dr. Sutton said it wasn't until the 1950s that scientists discovered that it wasn't the growth hormone itself that increased growth. It seems that hGH stimulates production of growth factors known as somatomedins which are secreted in the liver and other organs. Not until the 1960s was a test developed to measure the concentration of human growth hormone in human plasma.

The secretion of human growth hormone is altered by exercise, with the extent of the alteration dependent on the duration and intensity of the exercise. More intense exercise causes higher levels of hGH to be secreted and accumulated in the plasma.

Severe imbalances of hGH cause marked aberrations. The absence of natural hGH secretion will cause an individual to be a dwarf (unless he is treated). Too much hGH, on the other hand, causes a condition known as acromegaly, in which there is overgrowth. It is most noticeable in the face and hands, but also occurs in internal organs. Very large and prominent bones in the face, enlargement of the fingers and toes, and coarsening of the skin are common characteristics. A person with acromegaly may also develop diabetes, heart or thyroid disease. Menstrual disorders occur in women, and sexual interest may decrease in both sexes.

We know little about the side effects of hGH in healthy athletes except that they are at risk for developing acromegaly. Until 1985, athletes' access to the drug was more limited. Then Genentech put Protropin on the market and sales reached nearly $44 million in 1986. Eli Lilly and Company put its product, Humatrope, on the market in 1987. There have been thefts and diversions at both places, although security procedures are strict.

One reason for medical interest in hGH is because some researchers believe there may be a role for hGH in treating osteoporosis and obesity, although it hasn't been proven clinically effective for either condition yet.

There is no test yet to detect the presence of excess human growth hormone, but it is on the list of banned drugs. An FDA spokesman said he has seen reports of athletes taking megadoses of the drug, up to 20 times the recommended dosage, and said the public should be aware of the drug's very serious side effects. It was believed that the cost and impurity of the black market supply would keep the number of athletes using hGH low for the immediate future, but there are reports that its use is increasing. If doctors are persuaded to prescribe the drug for people who simply want to be taller, it may set an unfortunate precedent. For instance, nobody knows how many professional basketball players may have taken the drug, but we can see that players the world over are getting taller. Seven-foot players are no longer a rarity.

BLOOD DOPING by U.S. cyclists was a scandal of the 1984 Olympic Games in Los Angeles. Several cyclists admitted having participated in this practice which, strictly speaking, does not involve drug use at all.

Blood doping is a process by which blood is withdrawn from the body, frozen for the time it takes the body to rebuild its own red cell supply, and then thawed and reinfused before a competition. Cyclists must have endurance, and the history of this sport includes the use of many drugs to boost endurance. When drug testing was instituted, blood doping replaced amphetamines as the illicit performance enhancer of choice.

This is the theory behind blood doping: Red blood cells carry oxygen to exercising muscles. If you have more red blood cells than the other guy, you should be able to do more work because energy metabolism is most efficient when the oxygen supply is abundant. Blood doping is useful only for endurance sports, or aerobic exercise. In anaerobic exercise, where an athlete does short bursts of work such a lifting a heavy weight or throwing a discus, a continuous supply of oxygen isn't critical.

The percentage of red blood cells in the blood is called the hematocrit, and normal people have a hematocrit of about 40 to 45 percent. Plasma makes up the rest of the blood. Suppose you boost your hematocrit to 50 percent. Then an extra 5 to 10 percent of red cells are available to carry oxygen. Dr. Wadler and Dr. Hainline say in their book that an athlete's total blood volume circulates five to six times each minute in maximal exercise. An athlete could increase the potential extra oxygen available to his tissues by about 0.5 liters per minute.

Athletes may think that if a little is good, a whole lot is better, but that thinking can be dangerous when you change the composition of blood. The red cells also make blood thicker so that it moves more slowly and clots more easily.Dr. Wadler and Dr. Hainline note that this forces the heart to work much harder to move the thickened blood, causing the blood pressure to rise and exercise capacity to decrease. The body has a natural compensating mechanism for handling an increased volume of red cells. Plasma is shifted from within the vessels out into the tissues so that the actual blood volume in the body remains at a normal level even if it is somewhat thicker, they say.

The way blood doping works is relatively simple, although athletes must have assistance in withdrawing, storing, and reinfusing the blood. Anywhere from four to 12 weeks before a competition, two pints of blood are removed from the body and the red cells separated from the plasma and preserved by freezing. (It is possible to preserve the blood by refrigeration but then it can only be held for about three weeks and it takes an athlete longer than three weeks to regain his former hemoglobin level.) After the blood is withdrawn, the athlete continues to train while his body replenishes its blood supply. Sometime between one and seven days before competition, the frozen red cells are thawed and added to a salt solution and reinfused into the body, a process that takes a couple of hours.

Athletes may think that if a little is good, a whole lot is better, but that thinking can be dangerous when you change the composition of blood.

Studies have supported the belief that blood doping can increase endurance, perhaps as much as 25 percent, depending upon an individual athlete's level of aerobic fitness. The main dangers to health are in the withdrawing and reinfusing process. Although nearly all blood doping is done by the process described above, some athletes have used red cells from a donor with the same blood type and who is a close match. However, this process always carries an increased health risk, including the possibility of transmitting AIDS.

ERYTHROPOIETIN is a hormone normally produced by the kidneys that stimulates bone marrow to produce red blood cells. Recombinant DNA techniques have permitted scientists to manufacture erythropoietin in the laboratory, and the Food and Drug Administration has approved the sale of this drug to treat patients who have anemia because of kidney disease. There have been remarkable results from using erythropoietin for very ill patients; in one trial, it eliminated the need for transfusions and restored normal hematocrit. In the future, erythropoietin may be used for patients who are less seriously ill, but for now, the potential U.S. market is less than 30,000 people, and treatment is expensive, approximately $6,000 a year.

There is no indication for erythropoietin use in healthy people. However, there can be no doubt that erythropoietin (EPO) is THE hot drug for endurance athletes. Over the past two years, seven bicycle racers from the Netherlands have died either during races or shortly after completing them, and there is a strong suspicion that EPO may be involved. The Royal Dutch Cycling Federation announced in March 1990 that it is investigating possible stimulant abuse. A U.S. drug expert said he has been told that the use of EPO is rampant among marathon runners, both men and women.

Hematologists report being questioned by athletes who see it as an easier and more effective way to blood dope. Instead of going through the withdrawing, freezing, thawing, and reinfusing that must be done with real blood, using erythropoietin just involves a series of injections. The athlete's own bone marrow would get to work turning out red cells. The potential problem is that, like the Sorcerer's Apprentice, the bone marrow might keep cranking out red cells if the erythropoietin dosage is misjudged.

As the hematocrit goes up, the blood thickens, and at a certain point, which many hematologists think is a hematocrit of 55 percent or greater, an element of danger is present. Moreover, endurance athletes, the very people most tempted to try erythropoietin, often have elevated hematocrits at the end of a race anyway because of the fluid loss they sustain during competition.

John Dipersio, M.D., a hematologist, told colleagues at UCLA that the potential for driving the hematocrit dangerously high exists with erythropoietin. "Anyone who runs a marathon loses a tremendous amount of water," Dr. Dipersio has said. "In an Olympic marathon, a male runner might begin the race with a hematocrit of 42 percent or 43 percent. With an outdoor temperature of 50 to 55 degrees, he might finish with a hematocrit of 55 percent because of fluid loss."

There is no indication for erythropoietin in healthy people. However, there can be no doubt that erythropoietin (EPO) is THE hot drug for endurance athletes.

What is left is, in Dr. Dipersio's words "sludging red cells." Take the same marathon runner and give him erythropoietin so that he begins the race with a hematocrit anywhere from 52 to 58 percent. By race end, his hematocrit could be in the high 60s. That could be very dangerous, perhaps leading to a heart attack, stroke, heart failure, or pulmonary edema. Moreover, the danger doesn't necessarily end when the race does. The hematocrit may continue to rise for five or 10 days after the last injection. A marathoner who has his last injection two days before a race may be at risk for three to seven days afterward. Hematologists and sports medicine specialists warn that there could be deaths from using erythropoietin. It may have already happened.

Because it is so new, nothing is known about its use in athletes or availability on the black market.

AMPHETAMINES were widely used by athletes and nonathletes alike from the late 1940s until 1970, with the high point in the 1960s. They were developed in the 1930s and used during World War II by both German and American soldiers to prevent fatigue. Such diverse groups as college students and truck drivers have made use of amphetamines. In sports, they have been favored by endurance and strength athletes, cyclists, runners, and professional football players. Amphetamines are on the banned drug lists because they may enhance speed, power, endurance, concentration, and fine motor coordination.

Two events caused amphetamine use to plunge sharply. First, they became scheduled drugs when the Controlled Substances Act of 1970 was passed by Congress. This means there are strict guidelines for their medical use. Second, drug testing virtually wiped out the use of amphetamines in the Olympic sports because they must be used at the time of competition. Undoubtedly, there is still some use among athletes who don't face drug testing in their sports.

BETA BLOCKERS are heart drugs, used to treat high blood pressure, exertional heart pain, and irregularities of heart rhythm. They have become popular because one of their effects is to relieve anxiety and stage fright. Their antianxiety properties are the basis of their use by athletes and the reason they are banned drugs. In sports like shooting and archery where steadiness is important, beta blockers could give an athlete an edge. However, they can be detected by drug testing.

DIURETICS are drugs that promote increased urination and give a small but rapid weight loss. These drugs have been favored by wrestlers and others who must compete in specified weight classes. Jockeys and gymnasts have also used them. Another reason athletes might turn to diuretics is to reduce the concentration of other drugs — like anabolic steroids — in the urine by diluting them in the increased amount of urine. However, now diuretics are also on the banned drug lists and can be detected by drug testing.

Questionable Practices

SODA LOADING refers to the practice of consuming a large quantity of baking soda before competing, in the belief that it serves to buffer the lactic acid buildup in the muscles that causes fatigue. Presumably, this would help anaerobic events like sprinting. There is some question about whether this practice enhances sports performance, but large amounts can cause diarrhea and gastric distress and hurt performance.

AMINO ACIDS are substances in the blood formed when dietary protein is broken down by enzymes in the digestive tract. According to Dr. Wadler and Dr. Hainline, athletes believe that taking in extra amino acids in the form of commercially produced pills helps increase muscle bulk or energy utilization, and stimulates the release of growth hormone within the body. For whatever reason, these dietary supplements sell briskly. However Dr. Wadler and Dr. Hainline also note that amino acid supplements have never been shown to benefit endurance athletes or bodybuilders who are in good health and who eat a well-balanced diet. They rarely are taken in excessive amounts because of the cost, but large quantities could cause liver and kidney damage, dehydration, excessive loss of urinary calcium, and mental disturbance.

VITAMINS AND MINERALS are believed by many athletes to be absolutely necessary to maintaining top physical form. Like amino acid supplements, vitamins and minerals are purchased regularly and in large quantities. Vitamins are needed to maintain normal metabolic cell function, according to Dr. Wadler and Dr. Hainline, but they see no reason to add them to a well-balanced diet. Having extra vitamins and minerals in the body has not been shown to improve strength, increase endurance, improve peak running speed, improve VO2max, or blood lactate turnpoint, the doctors say. There is plenty of evidence in the medical literature to show that excessive vitamin intake can cause disorders, and that overdoses of vitamins can be potentially serious.

Enhancing Physical Performance Legally

As we said as the beginning, a good night's rest can make a big difference in how a given athlete performs. The way an athlete prepares himself physically for his competition can make the difference between success and failure. Some of these successful preparation techniques that enhance physical performance are available to anyone who wants to study and practice them, or to seek out the aid of experts. They carry no risk to health and actually improve it in most instances. Athletes who use these techniques and practices may gain an edge over those who don't, but they are not cheating, merely maximizing their natural ability.

NUTRITION is one of the easiest performance enhancing factors to control. Most of the ancient attempts to optimize sports performance focused on eating certain foods. Getting the best effect from nutrition requires long-range planning, preferably with an expert in the field. Several professional sports teams employ nutritional consultants. Examples of dietary manipulations include maintaining adequate fluid intake and proper selection of precompetition meals. Sports nutrition has not been as well studied in the U.S. as it has in some other countries, and this is an area where we can expect to see continued development.

WEIGHT TRAINING is another form of conditioning that is available to all athletes although it is more difficult and less obvious than it seems. Properly done, it can significantly improve sports performance. Before embarking on intensive weight training, athletes should undergo a program of general physical conditioning to improve their strength and flexibility. Specific elements in any weight training program should be developed by someone familiar with the demands of the sport so that the training is sports specific. A football player would not expect to have the same weight training program as a swimmer or a gymnast, but all three can benefit.

BIOMECHANICS is one of the most promising and interesting areas of sports performance. By breaking a given sports activity down into its component parts and studying the mechanical activities required to perform it, an athlete can be shown how to achieve optimum results. A computer at the swimming research laboratory at the U.S. Olympic Center in Colorado Springs, can convert pictures of actual swimming strokes into stick figure representations. Physiologists study these to pinpoint areas where stroke improvement is possible. Another aspect of biomechanics is investigating the stresses placed upon the body during performance of a given sport. For example, orthopedic surgeons have learned a lot about knees in recent years, including the mechanics of how they give way under stress. By charting the patterns of movement and the way injuries occur, they gain information that is immediately useful in treating knee injuries and in designing equipment to help prevent injury.

EXERCISE PHYSIOLOGY is a field that covers exercise and fitness, and the processes involved in physical performance.When there is increased understanding of these processes, better training programs can be designed. Physiological testing of athletes has become very sophisticated and often involves physiologists and physicians working together to overcome problems that have impaired past performances. Nancy Hogshead, a former Olympic swimmer, wonders if her lack of knowledge may have cost her a gold medal. Hogshead always attributed her breathing problems to having small lungs until just after her Olympic race. A physician walked up to her on deck and said, "I think you have asthma." Exercise-induced asthma is a common but treatable condition if it is recognized. Still another aspect of exercise physiology is the study of how athletes adapt to changes in climate and time zones. This can be very important to individuals who compete all over the world. A tennis player might be in Australia one week and the U.S. the next, going from winter to summer weather in the process. What effect does that have on his or her game?

SPORTS MEDICINE is a growing area and one that is becoming increasingly sophisticated. Many athletes in many different sports are competing today after recovering from what would have been career-ending injuries only 10 or 20 years ago. Professional football players commonly undergo arthroscopic surgery on their knees or shoulders in the off season and come back to play again. Dan Hampton of the Chicago Bears has had 10 knee surgeries! Olympic and World Cup champion skier Phil Mahre had his greatest victories after being successfully treated for a shattered bone in his leg. Overtraining is a common cause of athletic injury, and specialists can manage many of these overuse problems. Most large metropolitan areas now have sports medicine specialists who have combined a knowledge of medicine and exercise physiology to help athletes achieve maximum potential.

Psychological Performance Enhancement

Sports psychology, although still considered a "soft" science by many sports scholars, is one of the fastest growing areas of research. At a 1989 conference in Colorado Springs sponsored by the International Olympic Committee, an entire section of the meeting was devoted to sports psychology.

All athletes know that the effects of the mind on the body can be quite dramatic. What many athletes refer to as "getting up" for an athletic event means achieving an optimum mental state of arousal, a state that Dr. Wadler and Dr. Hainline characterize as covering such terms as alertness, stress, wakefulness, excitement, concentration, attention, drive, and motivation. Low levels of arousal are associated with poor performance and are a major reason for sports "upsets." Arousal is not, however, entirely under the voluntary control of an athlete. This complex state cannot be summoned at will. Moreover, athletes sometimes become overaroused before competing and feel tense, angry, frustrated, or even panic-stricken, according to Dr. Wadler and Dr. Hainline. It is a delicate balance but when optimal arousal is achieved at the time of athletic performance, athletes report being unaware of their surroundings, feeling neither fatigue or pain, experiencing perceptual changes such as time slowing down or objects becoming larger, and feeling unusual power and control. Records are set and games are won during periods of optimal arousal.

Stress is a word that has two meanings in sports, one good and one bad. Stress may promote that state of readiness to compete that is called arousal and which must be present in any successful athletic performance, or it can be a debilitating state that prevents an athlete from doing his or her best. Dr. Wadler and Dr. Hainline have noted that what may be positive stress (eustress) for one athlete can be negative (distress) for another. Stress, they say, often shows itself as anxiety, but anxiety is related to motivation and appears to be the internal energizer that supports goal-directed behavior. Many successful athletes are intense, ambitious people who drive themselves beyond ordinary limits. The trick is not to let the anxiety get out of control so that it slips from eustress to distress.

A number of psychological techniques have been developed to handle stress and promote arousal, and these have been discussed by Dr. Wadler and Dr. Hainline in their book. Briefly, they include:

BIOFEEDBACK is a process that teaches an athlete to consciously control the physiological components of the stress response. With the help of electronic instruments, he learns to recognize when the heart rate or muscle tension is increasing. Biofeedback is an apparently useful tool.

GOAL SETTING simply refers to the practice of identifying what an individual hopes to gain from a sports performance and what steps must be taken to achieve those gains. If there is a long-term goal, setting intermediate goals is advisable. There is a great deal of evidence that setting goals is beneficial to task performance.

RELAXATION TRAINING refers to being able to relax the nervous system and muscles at will. The effect is to keep muscles from becoming overtense at the time of competition. Deep breathing may also be used to achieve a relaxation response. Relaxation training will enhance concentration, relaxation, and optimize muscle metabolism. An athlete who is relaxed will have a fluidity of movement and be able to maintain a relaxed, but aroused state, giving him an edge over competitors whose muscles are tense.

ASSERTIVENESS TRAINING is a technique that focuses on the behavioral and cognitive aspects of the stress response. It has been used to help athletes who may fear disapproval or anger or who are anxious when they interact with teammates or coaches. It also can help athletes who respond with inappropriate anger when they are faced with a situation where they cannot control the outcome. It requires thinking positively, maintaining self-control, and being goal-oriented.

IMAGERY AND MENTAL PRACTICE is a technique espoused by many athletes, including Leigh Ann Fetter, the University of Texas swimmer who holds the 50-meter record for women. This technique involves visualizing the competition before it actually occurs, and it apparently is a more effective training method for athletes in individual sports than for those in team sports where the actions of others cannot be controlled or consistently predicted. However, swimmers like Fetter can "preswim" the whole race in their heads, imagining the start, stroke technique, turn, and sprint to the finish. Such visualization may activate the neurological and physiological pathways that are associated with actually performing the activity. There are some questions about the effectiveness of this technique but Fetter and others are convinced it works.

SELF TALK refers to the practice of making mental self-statements that direct attention to the performance at hand and which repudiate negative thoughts. An athlete who dwells on negative past performance can hurt his or her chances of performing well the next time, but replacing those negative thoughts with positive statements, may enhance the next performance. In a nutshell, this is the power of positive thinking.

PSYCHOLOGICAL COUNSELING is an avenue that may be used when an athlete is unable to overcome a situation independently. Sports psychologists can identify factors that prevent an athlete from achieving his or her potential, and give advice on dealing with them appropriately. Mike Tomczak, quarterback of the Chicago Bears, got psychological counseling to help him deal with volatile, mercurial coach Mike Ditka and, indeed, it was obvious the next season that he had become more assertive and self-confident. Elite athletes may have a regular sports psychologist. One word of caution: carefully check the credentials of a sports counselor before entering treatment since this is a new and growing field which has not always been well regulated.

9

THE LAST WORD

The previous eight chapters have been grounded in fact, either based on research or expert opinion. This last chapter is an essay about what we and others see as the root causes of the problem with anabolic-androgenic steroids and our views on what action we believe is needed.

All illicit drug taking probably has some of the same root causes. Both recreational and performance-enhancing drugs produce *altered states* of mind and body. Steroids are more likely to be viewed as "upwardly mobile drugs," or "success oriented drugs." There probably is some small overlap in the user groups, although many steroid users never touch other drugs, not even alcohol.

In our view, some important root causes are:

- The belief that drugs can solve problems
- Too much pressure for conformity
- According athletes special treatment
- The belief that winning is the only worthwhile goal

It would be nice to say that we are hopeful that the proposed federal legislation to control steroids would work, or that the stepped up enforcement campaign would solve this drug problem. However, the greatest impact on lessening the use of performance enhancement drugs would come from revising our attitudes toward the importance of physical appearance and of "winning." It is in that context that sports and athletes become much more than games of skill played by physically strong and talented people.

So long as such extraordinary emphasis is placed on winning, and sports contests are so important to society, the incentives to use performance-enhancing drugs will outweigh any health or legal risks. Drugs will also continue to be attractive to men with a narcissistic personality type so long as we equate strength and power with masculinity.

Both recreational and performance-enhancing drugs produce altered states of mind and body.

This is a problem that will only grow as technology improves. Recently, we heard about two new types of performance-enhancing drugs that some athletes will undoubtedly be trying soon. For that reason alone, we must recognize the importance of drugs in our society.

Summing up the current situation with anabolic-androgenic steroids:

- There is widespread use of drugs that cause profound derangements of body chemistry that may not be entirely reversible.

- These drugs may cause serious behavior problems in an unknown number of users.

- Psychological dependence may occur.

- Immense doses — far beyond any therapeutic range — are common.

- Drugs purchased on the black market may pose health risks.

- Use of anabolic steroids may lead to the use of other drugs of various types.

- Aside from the potential physical, psychological, or moral repercussions, the use of these drugs can have serious legal consequences.

The Historical Perspective

It may come as a surprise to some, but Americans have a long history of drug use, and narcotics control has been a problem for more than 100 years. Looking at that history makes many experts wonder if there is something in the collective psyche that impels us to seek altered states of consciousness. One Harvard researcher has suggested that mood alteration is a primary drive of human beings and, if that is so, such behavior could not be easily extinguished. While anabolic steroids don't produce the euphoric effects that are seen with cocaine or marijuana, they do alter mood.

Medical historian David Musto, M.D., a Yale University psychiatrist, has tracked U.S. drug use patterns, and he notes that opium use was well established in the U.S. by the time of the Civil War.

Some soldiers became addicts through medical treatment with remedies that contained opium. Laudanum was a popular drug of the time, and Dr. Musto says it was concocted of opium dissolved in sherry and flavored with cinnamon, cloves, and saffron. Addicted veterans may have recruited other drug users. By the late 1800s, cocaine was also very popular as a general tonic, and it was prescribed as a "cure" for opium, morphine, and alcohol habits. Many "health tonics" of the period were loaded with harmful drugs. By the turn of the century, the U.S. had a comparatively large number of drugs addicts, perhaps as many as 25,000.

Looking at (our) history makes many experts wonder if there is something in the collective psyche that impels us to seek altered states of consciousness.

After 1900, the social climate changed and drug use came to be viewed as an offense against society. This posture was maintained until the next big wave of drug use in the 1960s. Now, after 25 years of fairly casual tolerance, the U.S. is again showing signs of adopting a stricter attitude toward some types of drug use.

Even so, we still obviously cling to the notion that drugs can and should be used to solve many of life's problems. An alien viewing American television commercials could easily get the impression that nature has dealt shabbily with humans who apparently need an endless array of over-the-counter drugs to enable them to cope: pain relievers, products for gastric distress, products to induce "regularity," or products to induce sleep.

That doesn't even include prescription drugs, a field where some of the discoveries have been little short of miraculous. However, like atomic energy, most of these drugs have both the power to help and the power to harm.

The current move to legalize recreational drug use is based on the theory that addicts could obtain their drugs safely and probably less expensively. Crimes associated with drug use would decline. Many respected Americans do not believe legalizing drugs would cause any increase in the number of people who misuse them. But when we see that our legal drugs — alcohol, tobacco, and caffeine — are used without restraint, legalization is not as attractive, particularly so long as we continue with the mind set that drugs solve problems.

Drugs not only fail to solve problems, they usually create more while making the user temporarily feel better, and disinclined to deal realistically with problems. Users of so-called recreational drugs usually are unable to be objective about the benefits. This may also be true of steroid users. Yet, almost one in 10 Americans used an illicit drug within the last month.

Using drugs to enhance athletic performance is simply a continuation of the practice of using drugs as problem solvers. If you are not heavy enough for your sport, take a drug. If you need more strength, drugs can help. In a high-tech society, anabolic-androgenic steroids are simply another tool. Well, perhaps not just another tool. Many experts say, and we agree, that the desire to be physically strong and powerful is very deep-rooted in the male mind.

Athletes don't put steroids in the same category as other illicit drugs. Elite athletes have always viewed steroids as an integral part of training to achieve personal excellence and competitive success. They don't believe for a moment that they are cheating; they are simply maximizing their potential.

When a strong belief that drug taking solves problems prevails in a society that wants and expects instant gratification, the result is a philosophy that success need not be the culmination of a long process of learning and training, but rather, can be reached quickly. Then we see exactly how attractive steroids can be. An athlete who wishes to compete undrugged at the elite level may sacrifice his chance of success.

Being Just Alike

A second reason for our drug problem is peer pressure, which was identified in a Home Box Office television program on drug abuse as the Number 1 cause. Why is peer pressure so powerful?

Conforming generally to the standards of the culture is important. People who can't conform at all often end up in jail or in mental institutions. However, conformity can be overdone. From the time the smallest children go to nursery school, the pressure to be alike is on, sometimes producing cookie cutter children. Some parents who value individuality seek out alternative systems that allow their children to make choices, but these alternatives are not available to everyone. The process of conformity accelerates in public school. Woe to a child that "sticks out" or is "different." Not only is he likely to experience ridicule and rejection by his peers, but teachers have been known to excuse this cruel behavior by saying that it is simply the nature of children.

We make these statements with apologies to the many fine teachers who do respect children as individuals, but we still believe that the overall public education emphasis is not on teaching tolerance but on teaching conformity. In its own way, U.S. society can be as rigid as the Asian societies, but we lack their values of respect for family and authority. The ideals and values of our own society have become blurred over the years so that the conformity that we inculcate is simply conformity to the peer group. At its most extreme end, we have pathological conformity like a Charles Manson group or the Jim Jones congregation.

Most peer group conformity never advances to such an aberrant stage, but it does cause many youngsters to engage in practices they know are wrong and which they really don't want to do. When our children reach puberty, we say to them, "Think for yourself," or "Just say no." Unless young people have been prepared to think and act as individuals all along, it will never happen. The power of the previous 13 to 15 years of conditioning may be simply too powerful to overcome.

Conditioning for conformity is not limited just to the children. The fear that a child might be rejected by his peer group is so strong in many parents that they forego common sense and permit behavior they know is harmful. A high school sports team celebrated winning the state championship with a private party at a home where there were no adult chaperones and where alcoholic beverages were available in abundance.

One woman, who planned to permit her 15-year-old daughter to attend, said, "She has to learn to be a part of the group."

When there is a lack of focus on moral and cultural values, situational ethics are produced. Then a parent or coach can reason like this: Sports are conducted like wars. Whatever physical and mental benefits there may be to participation are just side issues. Winning is the most important thing. Therefore, I am justified in doing whatever it takes to see that my child/team wins.

When there is a lack of focus on moral and cultural values, situational ethics are produced.

As we enter a new decade, there are at least 23 colleges in the U.S. on NCAA probation for cheating, and the figure has been even higher. During the 1980s, 57 out of 106 Division I schools were punished by sanction, censure, or reprimand. If Division II and III schools are added, more than 100 schools are on the list. Where were the trustees of these schools while this behavior was occurring? In many cases, they were turning a blind eye to the evidence. Sports has no lock on situational ethics; it extends to every aspect of American life. So we have industrial espionage, insider trading, falsifying research, compensation fraud, and other forms of cheating, much of it sanctioned by peer group example. This sends a very clear message to our youth that cheating is okay if you get away with it. The disgrace is in being caught.

Athletes as Special People

Over 20 million North Americans participate in some form of organized sports, with peak participation coming between the ages of 11 and 13. After that, there is a sharp and steady decline. Elite athletes make up only a fraction of those 20 million people. Fewer than 2 percent of athletes who play major college sports ever play professional sports. So we see that sports participation is a pyramid, with many at the bottom and only a few at the top. Yet, many parents give a lower priority to education than they do to sports because they have been taken in by what Charles Yesalis, Sc.D., at Pennsylvania State University, calls "the big lie."

Yet, many parents have given a lower priority to education than they do to sports because they have been taken in by "the big lie."

He defines "the big lie" as encouraging kids to made bad life decisions based on the prospects, which are actually slim to none, that they will play Division I football or in the NFL, be part of Major League Baseball, or become tennis or golf professionals, or Olympic athletes. Moreover, says Dr. Yesalis, the life of an athlete at the top often is not as satisfying as the public perceives it to be. NFL players have been known to say privately that they don't have fun at the football games anymore, and that they see them as what they do to make a living. They are careful not to publicize this view because they are supposed to be playing for love of the game. In any event, the average career span of an NFL player is only three and a half years. If no preparation has been made for a life after sports, the athlete suffers.

We have made athletes special people in our society, individuals who are singled out for favored status because of their physical gifts. This may have been true even when primitive humans were still divided into hunters and gatherers. Physical prowess brought recognition then. It still does. We have simply changed the reward structure and upped the ante for winning.

Special treatment of an athletically gifted child may begin at a young age and continue until the end of his sports career. They may be given the impression that they are exempt from ordinary responsibilities of courtesy and respect for others. Adults may comfort an eight-year-old who throws a tantrum on the tennis court because he lost and let his inappropriate behavior pass without comment. People still excuse John McEnroe's excesses by saying that he behaves as he does because he hates to lose, leaving the false impression that his opponents don't mind it so much.

We also excuse bad behavior in coaches. Sports announcers have even developed euphemisms to describe fits of temper. When Michigan football coach Bo Schembechler went into a rage at a nationally televised game, the sportscaster said, "He's a real competitor."

When little athletes compete at higher levels, they have limited time to spend with peers, and they get slighted on developing social and political skills. Some never have an opportunity to act independently until their sports careers are over. One ex-professional athlete said that despite spending years traveling on airplanes, he discovered he didn't know how to make an airline reservation on his own after his playing days were over.

This continual favored status has been very harmful to some athletes, turning them into one-dimensional people who are gifted physically but retarded emotionally and intellectually. This is by no means universal. Many top athletes are bright, funny, capable, energetic, compassionate people who have learned how to balance sports with public life, and how to resist pressures from people around them who want to use or manipulate them.

We have made athletes special people in our society, individuals who are singled out for favored status because of their physical gifts.

Another problem with the proliferation of elite sports programs for athletic youngsters is that they are forced to specialize early before their bodies are ready for the strains of elite competition. Lyle Micheli, M.D., a Boston orthopedic surgeon and past president of the American College of Sports Medicine, says that doctors see sports injuries, primarily from overuse, that were unknown several years ago. An example presented at the 1989 ACSM meeting was of a teen-age gymnast whose high level training had caused a disruption of the growth plate in her wrist. Knee injuries are very common in young runners and sometimes these youthful knees sustain permanent damage.

Over the course of his interscholastic and collegiate sports career, an athlete must continually balance the demands of his career and academic life. College football players are sometimes disparaged for not making more of their academic opportunities but many say that Division I football is a full-time job in itself. It becomes harder for them not to look upon some special privileges as payment for doing a good job. Parking tickets or speeding violations are "overlooked," final examinations are adjusted, new clothes or perhaps a new car are available. Drinks and dinner at a restaurant are on the house. A dark side of escalating special treatment that comes with recognition of athletic talent is that many of the gifts and privileges have strings attached as others seek to tie themselves to public figures.

Nearly all elite athletes will be offered drugs at some point in their careers, either drugs to help them "celebrate" or to relax, or drugs to help them enhance their athletic performance. Because most athletes are young and in the stage of life where risk-taking behavior is normal, many take the risk.

We're Number 1

If an athlete is offered drugs to help him perform better, and if he is reasonably sure his drug use won't be discovered, he may find it hard to say no. He probably is well aware that in our society, if you don't win, you're a loser. Moreover, we espouse the notion that winning is more important than playing fair. You may be the second best miler in your state, the runner-up in the Super Bowl, the third best Little League team in the country, but you're still a loser. This type of thinking is strongly reinforced by the winner-take-all pattern of financial and emotional compensation. Losing a fair competition where an athlete has done his best should never be cause for regret or shame.

Let's take a moment to point out that not all athletes operate under the same pressures. Athletes in the money sports in Olympic competitions or in professional sports experience great pressure and are highly visible. When track star Carl Lewis attended a press conference in Washington, D.C. last October, he advanced into the room preceded, followed, and flanked by reporters and cameramen. Only in sports that have little commercial value attached to a gold medal can we still find athletes competing for the sheer joy of being the best they can be. Greg Barton won a gold medal in Seoul in kayaking just as Lewis did in track. Barton is regarded as the finest male kayaker the U.S. has produced, and he is a genuinely nice young man with a university degree and a profession. The will to meet the highest sports challenge is undoubtedly the same in both Barton and Lewis, but the reward structure is very different.

If the personal satisfaction from sports competition is derived from performing well, then all sports are important. A high school team winning a football game should have no higher value than an individual winning a noontime racquetball game, according to one drug expert.

The Role of Education

Education surely offers the best hope for dealing with drug use by athletes and with the overinflated value we have placed on sports. The next question is what type of education will be most effective?

"Education directed to the user should be a low priority," says Penn State's Yesalis. "If I had a million dollars to spend on education, I'd put

$900,000 of it into reaching parents and teachers, not necessarily to tell them how to recognize when a kid is using performance enhancement drugs, but to tell them that kids use these drugs because of the way we raise them. If you were stranded on a desert island, you might use cocaine if it were available, but nobody would use steroids. On a desert island, nobody cares what you look like and there is nothing to win. We are the ones who have made the determination that appearance and winning are all important. We're telling kids in our society that sports are more than a game. Until we change those signals, for the most part we might as well tell people to get used to drug use."

"We're telling kids in our society that sports are more than a game. Until we change those signals, for the most part we might as well tell people to get used to drug use.

Dr. Yesalis says he does support informing young people about what is known about the harmful effects of using anabolic-androgenic steroids and adds that he would like to see additional funds for research and drug testing. Research in which Dr. Yesalis participated showed that many steroid users would stop, if they had conclusive proof that there are lasting harmful effects. (It should also be noted that a small percent of those surveyed said they didn't care what research showed; they would not stop using the drugs.)

It seems to be true that when people use drugs, their perceptions about drugs change as they become part of a drug-related culture and seek out the company of other users. Traditional values that make a person feel good about himself, values such as dignity, integrity, honesty, and respect for others, are eroded and sometimes replaced by goals such as having power over others, notoriety, and money. Teenagers are particularly vulnerable because they are at a stage of life when they desire and need external approval. If society mandates strength, power, and skill at games as being very important, many of our youth will try to comply.

Young adults were not solely responsible for the actions that resulted in NCAA discipline for those 23 colleges on probation. Those violations were made by adults who were cheating the system, most often because the primary goal was to win and never mind how. Unless that attitude is revised, performance enhancement will continue to be a problem. The responsibility to stop corrupting sports contests rests with parents, coaches, teachers, athletic trainers, and fans as well as with athletes, and perhaps even more so.

Another part of education is learning how to help young people who are using anabolic steroids. Richard Strauss, M.D., editor-in-chief of *The Physician and Sportsmedicine*, says he believes that counseling is important.

"The only thing a doctor can really do," he says, "is see if they are healthy, so if you don't have some program available for them to redirect their energy, I don't think you will get very far."

Strauss says he thinks psychological dependency is not a problem for most young users, at least not in the same way that marijuana might be.

"However," he continued, "they do get hung up on it for social reasons. They like to be big and hang around the gym looking big. Then they find when they don't take the drug, they can't keep up the bulk and they get upset. You could call it a social addiction."

He advises parents to talk with a doctor who has had some experience with steroids, and to try to match a young user up with a drug counselor who is willing to tailor a program to the needs of the individual.

Looking to the Future

It seems clear to us that simply attacking the use of anabolic-androgenic steroids on the basis of health or ethical grounds will not produce the desired results unless there are changes in how we view athletes and sports competitions. It has been disheartening to see how many people have heaped praise on Ben Johnson for "his courage in coming forward," when that praise is undeserved. Johnson is, however, a victim of the system.

The question then becomes one of deciding what steps need to be taken to establish a societal context where taking performance-enhancing drugs will not be important. Dr.Yesalis has given some thought to how this should be done and he has made the following recommendations:

At the college level: *Eliminate athletic scholarships and give only merit scholarships, have random unannounced drug testing throughout the year, direct all university donations to the general fund, require equal sharing of television and bowl revenues, and establish tenure tracks for coaches.*

At the high school level: Eliminate television coverage of high school athletic events, limit the season length and the number and length of practices, increase the rewards for recognition of academic achievement, insist that attention is focused on personal excellence and not on winning, provide more resources for intramural sports, and conduct the hiring and firing of coaches on criteria other than win / loss records.

At the elementary level: Eliminate competitive sports for grade school children and replace them with lifetime fitness training and games, educate parents and coaches to focus on personal excellence, and eliminate football for this age group and alter Little League baseball.

We agree with many of Yesalis' suggestions. It was disconcerting to read recently that there is a ranking system for high school basketball players and that all college coaches know who's coming up — not just seniors, mind you, but all the way down to the freshman level. That's very daunting to a lot of youngsters who haven't yet found their game (but who will), and it gives the stars of the system the message that they have a lock on a career. Too often, such a system holds out false hope and puts kids on the road to ignoring education for false hopes of glory, or as Dr. Yesalis says: "We put kids on a pedestal for being good at what are really goofy games. We say that athletic skill is equal in importance with education, with making contributions to society, and with taking care of our families."

Medicine and science need to work together to bridge the gulf of mistrust between athletes and doctors. These two groups should be allies, not adversaries. There are some hopeful signs in that direction. There have been two national consensus conferences on anabolic-androgenic steroids, one of them in Rockville, Maryland, and the other in Los Angeles. There were problems with both meetings, but they were good first steps. Now it is time for a national organization or coalition of organizations to sponsor a steroid conference that serves as a forum to disseminate information and to agree on policy. Such a meeting should be open to the all those with an interest in the field. We are beyond the point where private scientific meetings about steroids are appropriate. Science and sport need to work together to solve the problems, and athletes and doctors need to trust one another again.

Physical contests can be fun, they can be sad, and they can be inspiring. What we don't want them to become is inhuman.

It will take the cooperation of medicine, science, and sports to maintain the integrity of what athletics should be in our lives, the development and exercise of physical excellence. There is beauty in athletic feats performed with skill and grace, and we admire the technical expertise. There is pride in seeing athletes achieve higher levels than they ever dreamed they could reach. It is uplifting to see human physical excellence at its best. Physical contests can be fun, they can be sad, and they can be inspiring. What we don't want them to become is inhuman.

MASTER SOURCE LIST

Brower, K.J. "Rehabilitation for Anabolic-Androgenic Steroid Dependence." Presented at the National Consensus Meeting on Anabolic-Androgenic Steroids, July 1989, Los Angeles, California.

Buckley, W.E., Yesalis, C.E., Friedl, K., Anderson, W., Streit, A., and Wright, J. "Estimated Prevalence of Anabolic Steroid Use Among Male High School Seniors." *Journal of the American Medical Association.* 1988, Vol 260:23.

Clinical Workshop on Drug Use and Abuse in Athletics, presented at the American College of Sports Medicine meeting, May 1989, Baltimore, Maryland.

Cowart, V.S. "Would Controlled Substance Status Affect Steroid Trafficking?" *The Physician and Sportsmedicine.* 1987, Vol 15:5.

Cowart, V.S. "Human Growth Hormone: The Latest Ergogenic Aid?" *The Physician and Sportsmedicine.* 1988, Vol 16:3.

Cowart, V.S. "Issues of Drugs and Sports Gain Attention as Olympic Games Open in South Korea." *Journal of the American Medical Association.* 1988, Vol 260:11.

Cowart, V.S.: "Erythropoietin: A Dangerous New Form of Blood Doping?" *The Physician and Sportsmedicine.* 1989, Vol 17:8.

Cowart, V.S. "Support Lags for Research on Steroid Effects." *Journal of the American Medical Association.* 1989, Vol 262:18.

Cowart, V.S. "Sports Medicine." In Medical and Health Annual. 1990, Encyclopedia Britannica, Inc., Chicago.

Dayton, L. "What Price Glory?" *Women's Sport & Fitness,* March 1990.

Di Pasquale, M.G. *Drug Use and Detection in Amateur Sports.* 1984 MGD Press, Warkworth, Ontario, Canada.

Feeling Good and Doing Better: Ethics and Nontherapeutic Drug Use. Hastings Center Report, 1984 Humana Press, Clifton, New Jersey.

Goldstein, P.J. "Anabolic Steroids: An Ethnographic Approach." Presented at the National Institute of Drug Abuse seminar, February 1989, Rockville, Maryland.

Hoberman, J. and Todd, T. "Heptathlete's Death Reflects Abuses in Sports Medicine." *Austin American-Statesman.* Sunday, October 4, 1987.

Hoberman, J. and Todd, T. "Pregnancy Doping: Female Athletes Confront Price of High Performance." *Austin American-Statesman.* Sunday, October 23, 1988.

Kashkin, K.B. and Kleber, H.D. "Hooked on Hormones?" *Journal of the American Medical Association.* 1989, Vol 262:22.

Kochakian, C.D. *Anabolic-Androgenic Steroids.* 1976, Springer-Verlag, New York.

Lamb, D.R. "Anabolic Steroids in Athletics: How Well Do They Work and How Dangerous Are They?" *American Journal of Sports Medicine.* 1984, Vol 12:1.

Lombardo, J. "Spotting the Young Steroid Abuser." *Diagnosis.* 1988, Vol 10:3.

Murray, T.H. "The Coercive Power of Drugs in Sports." The Hastings Center Report, August 1983.

National Institute of Drug Abuse Seminar, February 1989, Rockville, Maryland.

Pope H. and Katz D. "Affective and Psychotic Symptoms Associated With Anabolic Steroid Use." *American Journal of Psychiatry.* 1988, Vol 145

Pope, H. and Katz, D. "Homicide and Near-Homicide by Anabolic Steroid Users." *Journal of Clinical Psychiatry.* January 1, 1990.

Time. Health Section, January 8, 1990.

Strauss, R.H. *Drugs & Performance in Sports.* 1987, W.B. Saunders Company, Philadelphia.

Taylor, W.N. *Hormonal Manipulations: A New Era of Monstrous Athletes.* 1985, McFarland & Company, Inc., Jefferson, North Carolina, and London.

Telander, R. and Noden, M. "The Death of an Athlete." *Sports Illustrated,* Feb. 20, 1989.

Telander, R. "The Incredible Bulk." *Sports Illustrated.* April 24, 1989.

Underground Steroid Handbook, privately printed and circulated.

Wadler, G.I. and Hainline, B. *Drugs and the Athlete.* 1989, F.A. Davis Co., Philadelphia.

Wright, J.E. *Anabolic Steroids and Sports.* 1978, Sports Sciences Consultants, Box 555, N. Little Rock, AR 72115.

Wright, J.E. *Anabolic Steroids and Sports, Vol. II.* 1982, Sports Sciences Consultants, Box 555, N. Little Rock, AR 72115.

APPENDIX A: POSITION STANDS

A number of organizations have issued position stands on the use of anabolic-androgenic steroids by athletes. The U.S. Olympic Committee (USOC) and the National Collegiate Athletic Association (NCAA) have comprehensive drug policies and testing programs that cover but do not especially single out anabolic steroids.

The USOC bases its program on the stated premise that misuse of drugs by athletes "threatens the health of the athlete, the dignity of amateur sport, and public support of the Olympic movement." It maintains a complete drug testing program for the national governing bodies of the Olympic sports, so that each sport does not have to find and fund its own laboratory program.

The NCAA justifies its drug testing program for student athletes by saying that its testing program is "so that no one participant might have an artificially induced advantage, so that no one participant might be pressured to use chemical substances in order to remain competitive and to safeguard the health and safety of participants." It mandates drug testing for student athletes who compete in NCAA championships and postseason contests.

Below is a summary of the position stands on anabolic steroids of several organizations. Although they also have position stands on other drugs, we are covering only anabolic steroids. Those who are interested in knowing more about drugs policies of various organization will find a very comprehensive section on drug policies and position stands in the book *Drugs and the Athlete* by Gary Wadler, M.D., and Brian Hainline, M.D.

U.S. OLYMPIC COMMITTEE: The U.S.O.C.'s position is as follows: "These drugs are derivatives of the male hormone testosterone, which is also included in this banned class. They increase protein synthesis which may, with training, create an increase in lean muscle mass. This is perceived by athletes to increase strength and endurance. These drugs, being hormones, greatly interfere with the normal hypothalamic-pituitary-gonadal thermostat of hormonal balance. This interference in normal hormone function produces detrimental side effects."

AMERICAN COLLEGE OF SPORTS MEDICINE: Its stand on steroids contains the following points:

- Anabolic-androgen steroids in the presence of an adequate diet can contribute to increases in body weight, often in the lean mass compartment.

- The gains in muscular strength achieved through high-intensity exercise and proper diet can be increased by the use of anabolic-androgenic steroids in some individuals.

- Anabolic-androgenic steroids do not increase aerobic power or capacity for muscular exercise.

- Anabolic-androgenic steroids have been associated with adverse effects on the liver, cardiovascular system, reproductive system, and psychological status in therapeutic trials and in limited research on athletes. Until further research is completed, the potential hazards of the use of the anabolic-androgenic steroids in athletes must include those found in therapeutic trials.

Equitable competition and fair play are the foundation of athletic competition. If competition is to remain on this foundation, rules are necessary. The use of anabolic-androgenic steroids by athletes is contrary to the rules and ethical principles of athletic competition as set forth by many of the sports governing bodies. The American College of Sports Medicine supports these ethical principles and deplores the use of anabolic-androgenic steroids by athletes.

NATIONAL FOOTBALL LEAGUE: In its drug policy guide, the NFL says that misuse of anabolic steroids by NFL players has been impermissible ever since the League promulgated its policy on prescription drugs in the early 1970s. However, the League has gone a step further because of continuing use and says, "The League no longer merely condemns the misuse of these substances; they are prohibited in any quantity for any purpose." The League, which has done drug testing only once a year at the beginning of training camps, recently announced that players will be tested for steroids more frequently. A spokesman for the NFL said it is concerned about both the dangers of the drugs to the players who take them and the harm that might befall other players.

U.S. POWERLIFTING FEDERATION: In its drug control policy guide, the federation says that "using drugs to increase performance is intrinsically unfair" and that "support of amateur sports in the US by corporations and the public hinges on respectability and pride." With regard to anabolic steroids specifically, its says that increased injuries, including tendonitis and ruptured tendons and ligaments, are more likely to occur in athletes who use anabolic steroids.

In addition to these organizations, other sports governing bodies may include anabolic steroids on their lists of banned drugs or they may simply say, as does the policy of Major League Baseball, that there "is no place for illegal drug use in baseball" and that the use will not be condoned or tolerated. Some professional sports organizations prefer to keep details of any drug misuse by its athletes a private matter between the association and the player.

APPENDIX B: RESOURCES

Numerous organizations, both public and private, are developing materials and programs to address the problem associated with the abuse of performance-enhancing drugs. Those listed below are leading national organizations that have clearly and repeatedly demonstrated competence and commitment in this area.

THE AMERICAN COLLEGE OF SPORTS MEDICINE, probably the leading sports medicine organization in the world, has published position stands and opinion statements dealing with specific topics of interest to the scientific and lay communities (see Position Stands appendix). Although the recommendations are advisory only, the services of the ACSM are available to assist local and national organizations in implementing these recommendations. The position stands have become accepted policy by rules committees throughout the United States and in foreign countries. Copies of both the technical scientific position statements, as well as translations of these into a simplified lay format are available from the Public Relations Department, American College of Sports Medicine, Box 1440, Indianapolis, Indiana 46206-1440; (317) 637- 9200.

THE NATIONAL STRENGTH AND CONDITIONING ASSOCIATION has developed an action plan for coaches to identify and respond to the problem of anabolic steroid abuse among athletes. The plan and educational kit were developed by a select committee of renowned sports scientists and coaches to aid in instituting a school policy, providing understandable factual information on anabolic steroids, and establishing counseling and intervention guidelines. The kit is available free of charge to members of the association. Information about this program and the association is available from the National Strength and Conditioning Association, Box 81410, Lincoln, NE 68501; (402) 472-3000.

THE UNITED STATES OLYMPIC COMMITTEE has established a Drug Education Hotline (1-800-233-0393) which can provide information on drug testing, drugs that are approved for use in athletics, and drugs not approved for use in athletics. Educational materials have also been developed, including a video and guides to banned and safe medications. Materials can be obtained by calling the Hotline or contacting the U.S.O.C. Department of Library and Education Services, 1750 East Boulder Street, Colorado Springs, CO 80909.

TARGET, a service arm of the National Federation of State High School Associations, was founded in 1984 in response to the concern of alcohol and other drug use in schools across the nation. Because of TARGET's unique network with high schools through sports and activities, a significant database concerning steroids is maintained. In addition, TARGET has joined forces with the National Collegiate Athletic Association and the United States Olympic Committee to develop specific recommendations concerning the prevention of steroid use among amateur athletes. TARGET is a significant resource on education and prevention materials in the field of steroid and other drug use at the high school level. Information and materials may be obtained from: National Federation TARGET Program, P.O. Box 20626, Kansas City, MO 64195; (800) 366-6667.

THE U.S. FOOD AND DRUG AD-MINISTRATION has a major interest and responsibility with regard to the manufacturing, use, and effects of all drugs, including anabolic steroids and others used in performance enhancement. This organization has produced a variety of educational materials, including pamphlets, brochures, and posters, dealing with all illicit and abused drugs, including anabolic steroids. Materials and information can be obtained from or through the Consumer Affairs Department of the local district FDA office. The FDA also solicits the cooperation of athletes, coaches, and parents in providing information relating to the use, sources, or effects of these drugs, that might in any way be used to better protect the health of the public.

NARCOTIC AND DRUG RESEARCH, INC., is the largest and best-known non-profit corporation devoted to research and education in the drug abuse field. More than 200 staff members operate a research institute, a training institute, a resource center, and an AIDS outreach and prevention bureau. They have earned a world-wide reputation for their contributions to the overall understanding of the scope and nature of the drug abuse problem, its relationship to disease and crime, and to the improvment of drug abuse prevention and treatment. They offer numerous publications and more than 40 training programs on a variety of topics related to drug dependency, treatment, and prevention. In some 30 federal- and state-funded projects, they have demonstrated not only competence and capability but also dedication and commitment to communication and service that merits their inclusion in this section. NDRI is located at 11 Beach Street, New York, NY 10013; (212) 966-8700.

As a final note, videos are being marketed by a number of organizations, most of which seem to overstate or exaggerate the health risks involved with steroid use and abuse. These serve only to widen the gap of credibility and trust between athletes and the individuals who are responsible for their health and safety. It is advisable to screen videos for content before use rather than rely on advertising or other promotional materials. Two that are particularly noteworthy are *"Benny and the Roids"* from Disney Productions, which has garnered a number of awards from the National Education Association, and the newer and quite impressive *"What Price Glory? Myths and Realities of Anabolic Steroids"* from David Thomas Productions (561 Route 1, A2, Suite 169, Edison, NJ 08817), (800) 833-3270.

INDEX

Envopak system, 104
Epitestosterone, 111
Erythropoietin, 169-172
Esterification, 28-29, 30, 61-62
Esters of testosterone, 56, 106, 110, 112
Estrogen, 31, 67, 79
Ethical issues: 81, 139-158
Ethylestrenol, 7
Eunuchs, 19-20
Exercise physiology, 176
Fetter, Leigh Ann, 180
Food and Drug Administration (FDA), 119, 140, 166-167, 169-170, 209
Fibrocystic breast disease, 35, 55
Fitton, Tony, 123
Fluoxymesterone, 7
Flutie, Doug, 140
Football, 74, 75
Force platform, 149
Fowler, William, 43-44
Francis, Charlie, 153-154
Freitas, Luiz Batista, 119
Friedl, Karl, 59-61, 65, 111-112
Frost, Norman, 144, 145
Gas chromatography with mass spectroscopy (GC/MS), 105-107
Gender: differences in steroid effects, 20-21, 32-33, 47, 67, 70, 79-80, 147, 158
Genentech, 140, 166
Goal setting, 179
Goldman, Bob, 164
Goldstein, Paul, 82, 86, 89
Gynecomastia, 60
Hainline, Brian, 130, 160, 168, 173-174, 178-181, 203-204
Hair loss, 69, 74, 77
Hallucinations, 53
Hallucinogens, 126
Hampton, Dan, 177
Hasting on Hudson Center dialogue on drugs, 145-146
Hatfield, Frederick, 141-142
Heart problems, 62, 123, 171-172
Helmick, Robert, 101
Heroin, 126
Hervey, G.R., 42-43
High Technology Fitness Research Institute, 164
Hill, Jennifer, 132
Hoberman, John, 143-144, 146-147, 148-149, 157-158
Hogshead, Nancy, 176
Homewood-Flossmoor High School, 93-94, 98-99, 103, 108, 133
Homicide, 51-52
Hormones, 67; manipulation of, 143-144, 151; natural effects of, 22-25, 54-55, 77, 77-78
Hostility, 77-78
Human chorionic gonadotropin, 84

Human growth hormone, 2, 25, 162-167, 173; ethical issues surrounding use of, 139-141
Humatrope, 166
Hunter, John, 20
Hypertension, 65-66, 84, 172
Hypothalamus, 23-24
Hypothyroidism, 163
Imagery, 180
Immune system: as affected by steroids, 67
Infertility, 147
Informed consent, 156-158
Injectable anabolic steroids, 28 (list), 56, 106
International Amateur Athletic Federation, 156
International Olympic Committee (IOC), 97, 113, 130, 135, 137, 143, 160, 177; drug testing laboratories approved by, 96-97, 106, 107, 156, 164; medical commission, 108, 112
Jaundice, 80
Jenkins, David, 117-118
Johnson, Ben, 103, 109, 113-114, 119, 125, 153-155, 198
Jung, Carl, 150
Kammerer, R. Craig, 111
Kashkin, Kenneth B., 57-58
Katz, David L., 51-53
Kenyon, Alan, 34-35
Kidneys, 58, 169
Kleber, Herbert D., 57-58
Kochakian, Charles D., 21-22, 26, 129-130
Lamb, David R., 81-82, 122-123
Leggett, Don, 73-74
Leukemia, 163
Levine, Mel 125, 127
Lewis, Carl, 125, 195
Leydig cells, 25
Lilly, Eli and Company, 140, 166
Liothyronine sodium, 161
Liver: as affected by steroids, 58-62, 80; effects on testosterone, 26-27
Lombardo, John, 74, 75
Loyola University high school survey, 9
Luteinizing hormone (LH), 24
Mahre, Phil, 177
Malnutrition: steroid treatment of, 35
Mandarich, Tony, 142-143
Manic episodes, 53
Marijuana, 124
Masking agents, 106
McKeag, Douglas, 9-10, 63
McKeever, Barry, 132
Methandrostenolone, 29, 34, 52, 65
Methenolone, 52
Metabolism, 39
Metamphetamine, 126
Micheli, Lyle, 193